Merle Gr...

T0031759

Solace in the Storm

It's not every day that you come across such an empowering self-help book filled with incredible nuggets that are easy to digest and incorporate into everyday life as we care for our loved ones. No matter which stage of life you find yourself in as a caregiver, Dr. Merle Griff has written a road map to help guide you through what can be an overwhelming and complicated experience. Her book is beautifully written, peppered with positive and concise anecdotes that can be easily put into practice. As someone who sees both the direct as well as the indirect negative impacts that caring for a loved one can have in the workplace, both on the individual caregiver and the organization as a whole, I truly believe that the tools that Dr. Griff shares in her book can only serve to minimize what is typically a very disruptive time in their lives. I want to thank Dr. Griff for sharing her insights in such a genuine and meaningful light.

Andrew Bloom

President and chief executive officer
Corporate Synergies Group

A warm, wise, and (most importantly) practical resource for the many challenges facing today's families. Highly recommended!

Joshua Coleman, PhD

Psychologist and author
Rules of Estrangement: Why Adult Children Cut Ties and How to Heal the Conflict

Thanks to Dr. Griff for crafting a meaningful, moving, and motivational guide to caregiving. This is a resource readers will turn to again and again, as the lifespan approach connects us all as we progress along our caregiving journey.

Jed Johnson, MSW, MBA

Managing director, Aging Services
CARF National and International Accreditation Services

Dr. Merle Griff is a source of wise and practical guidance, with years of direct experience and professional education to back it up. What greater endorsement for a book about handling family situations could there be? The book offers not only useful knowledge and guidance but also a warmly engaging style that enables readers to readily understand and see how these insights can be applied to their own situations.

Karen VanderVen, PhD

Professor emerita
Department of Psychology in Education
University of Pittsburgh

Dr. Griff's professional and personal experiences have allowed me as the reader to better understand the multiple dynamics of caring and how to approach new situations. Caring requires a healthier, more capable caregiver. I know more now than I did before reading.

David Webb

Senior advisor and host
Veteran Services USA
The David Webb Show, Sirius XM: The Patriot Channel

I have known Dr. Merle Griff for several decades, and she is exceptionally insightful about the needs of family caregivers and those we care for. Merle combines her personal and professional experiences as she listens, learns, and focuses on the practical, actionable, and realistic takeaways that family caregivers so desperately need. This book will surely be a key resource for those who are caring for others.

Amy Goyer

Nationally known family caregiving expert
Author of *Juggling Life, Work, and Caregiving*

Solace *in the* Storm

MERLE GRIFF

Solace *in the* Storm

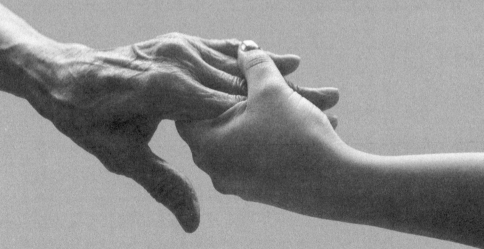

CARING FOR LOVED ONES
OF EVERY GENERATION

Forbes | Books

Published by Forbes Books, Charleston, South Carolina.
Member of Advantage Media.

Forbes Books is a registered trademark, and the Forbes Books colophon is a trademark of Forbes Media, LLC.

Printed in the United States of America.

10 9 8 7 6 5 4 3 2 1

ISBN: 979-8-88750-070-6 (Paperback)
ISBN: 979-8-88750-071-3 (eBook)

LCCN: 2023902364

Cover design by Megan Elger.
Layout design by David Taylor.

This custom publication is intended to provide accurate information and the opinions of the author in regard to the subject matter covered. It is sold with the understanding that the publisher, Forbes Books, is not engaged in rendering legal, financial, or professional services of any kind. If legal advice or other expert assistance is required, the reader is advised to seek the services of a competent professional.

Since 1917, Forbes has remained steadfast in its mission to serve as the defining voice of entrepreneurial capitalism. Forbes Books, launched in 2016 through a partnership with Advantage Media, furthers that aim by helping business and thought leaders bring their stories, passion, and knowledge to the forefront in custom books. Opinions expressed by Forbes Books authors are their own. To be considered for publication, please visit **books.Forbes.com**.

For my parents, whose love and care became my model for caring for others.

Contents

The Storm

Life can change in an instant. Suddenly, you can be thrown into the unfamiliar storm of caregiving.

That's what happened to me the day I got the call from my brother. He was in Florida, where he and my mother both lived. She had had a very dense stroke. Despite the best efforts of her doctors, the stroke took away her ability to speak, and she was paralyzed on one side.

But, as my friends always used to say, my mother's finger and her eyes could tell you a lot. Even though she wasn't speaking, she was still there. Rather than putting her in a nursing facility, I decided to bring her to live with me in Ohio.

Thus began my new life as her caregiver.

In actuality, I first became a caregiver as most people do: as a parent to my two sons. Despite my background as a therapist and expertise in working with children and families, I found new motherhood to be a challenge. Throughout those years, I learned a lot about the frustrations of that role and how overwhelming it could be.

Still, I wasn't prepared for how all consuming and stressful caring for my mother would be. I took care of her in my home for a number of years until she passed away. But that wasn't the end of my role as a caregiver. Not long after my mother died, my husband, who was retired, became ill and started to suffer from muscular weakness. He ended up in the hospital with double pneumonia and a type of flu that has a high fatality rate. He never recovered his strength. As I did with my mother, I kept him at home but this time with around-the-clock help. He was a large man, and I was not physically capable of moving him from bed to wheelchair or to perform all his personal care.

A few years later, I lost him after he contracted COVID-19 while in the hospital.

From parenthood, from caring for my mother and husband, and from listening to my clients, I've learned a lot about caregiving—lessons that you can't learn from a textbook. One thing I learned is that I didn't want to read a heavy textbook to get help! When you're overwhelmed, stressed, and have your hands full, you need ideas that are quick, easy, and digestible. Most information out there about caregiving is too long and takes too much time to read and then integrate into your life.

When I did a radio show on caregiving, I came to understand that you, as a family caregiver, need to hear something that you can take away, something that you can do in a couple minutes. We're talking about survival! That's the type of help I want to share with you.

And I also want you to understand, through the stories I share and from my own personal experiences, that others have been where you are now. Please know that you are not alone.

The Yin and Yang of Caregiving

Two lessons I've learned about caregiving can be found in this quote by Kahlil Gilbran:

> *Your living is determined not so much by what life brings to you as by the attitude you bring to life, not so much by what happens to you as by the way your mind looks at what happens.*[1]

I read this quote as saying that your life might be tough, you might have had a bad day, but you can always look at the same set of facts in two different ways. You can either continue to see things in a negative light, or you can reframe them to a positive.

For example, it's the difference between going to bed at night and thinking through how much the children annoyed you: "They drove me crazy today, and I'm exhausted." Or you can think along these lines: "I made it through the day. Someone else would not have done as well as I did. I'm a pretty good mom. The kids basically are healthy and doing well. We have enough money to live comfortably and have food on the table."

> 66
> Your living is determined not so much by what life brings to you as by the attitude you bring to life, not so much by what happens to you as by the way your mind looks at what happens.

There's a difference between those two ways of looking at things. Reframing like this can help.

---

1   Kahlil Gibran, quoted in Allison Carmen, *The Gift of Maybe: Finding Hope and Possibility in Uncertain Times* (New York: Penguin Group, 2014), 10.

On the other hand …

Caregivers sometimes need to feel the pain. You have to allow yourself to say, "This is a horrible thing that I'm going through. It's really, really difficult. I feel terrible about this, and it's hard for me."

And then you can move on.

Sometimes denying that emotion or reaction is doubly exhausting because you're experiencing it while denying it at the same time. Know that you're allowed to feel what you're feeling.

A Bit about Me

In addition to my life experience, I bring my background as a therapist to this topic. I began my professional career working with children and youths as a play therapist. I developed therapeutic techniques that have been published and used throughout the world, namely Family Play Therapy and Intergenerational Play Therapy. As director of the McKinley Center Intergenerational Project, I developed programs that brought together children—from babies through college age—with seniors.

In 1985, I founded the SarahCare Center, opening the first facility in Ohio. Originally called SARAH (Senior Adult Recreation and Health), the facility was one of the first intergenerational sites in the US. The senior adult day health center was located next to a child day care center and served as a training and research site for developing other unique intergenerational programs across the country.

A shift in our approach to caring for families and primary family caregivers was a result of my experience caring for my mother. I couldn't find suitable options for the families I worked with and for my own mother. That led me to expand SarahCare's services to include more programs designed to ease the stress of family caregivers and help them make their lives a little easier.

Have You Experienced These Situations?

I see some common patterns among caregivers and among their family members or friends who might want to help. Do any of these situations seem familiar? This book is filled with scenarios like these and practical feedback that you can put into action.

> *As a caregiver I must always strive to be understanding and patient, especially with members of my family who are seniors.*

While it might be acceptable to complain about your kids, there's a myth that you should always be kind and loving while caring for seniors and that they never do anything that would provoke you to be upset or to lose your patience with them. The myth is that the seniors are always pleasant, smiling, lovely people.

That's not true.

I've known seniors to take a cane and hit a family caregiver. I've known seniors to be very insulting and verbally abusive to a family caregiver.

The fact of the matter is they sometimes do things to provoke us and make us angry. It's acceptable to complain about it and to put a stop to these behaviors.

> *I am just doing what is expected of me. I shouldn't expect or look for gratitude or words of praise.*

I often deal with people who say, "I know I'm just a parent and that raising the kids is my job." Or "I know these are my parents, and I should be doing that because that's my responsibility. I shouldn't feel bad that no one ever says thank you to me or no one ever gives me a compliment."

That's not true either! It's okay to feel like you want approval, thanks, or appreciation. Don't hesitate to ask for it.

I understand that my family member who is providing care is tired and doing their best, but this is my parent also. And the care is not up to my standards. Even though I live in another city, it is my right to say whatever I feel needs to be said.

When you're caring for a relative such as a parent, family members (usually siblings) feel as though it's their right to walk in and say whatever they want when they're visiting. They immediately notice what they don't like and feel as though it's their right to say to the person who's been there, usually working and caregiving at the same time, "This is not right." They offer advice and tell you what you should be doing. But they're not the ones who are exhausted. They haven't been caregiving around the clock.

I try to say to siblings, you may be right in what you're saying, but everything will go a lot better if you open the door by saying something positive. There's always something positive that you can see and comment on. "Mom looks well fed. She looks happy." Or "She's dressed so nicely today. Thank you for taking care of her. What would we do without you?"

Say something that's positive at the beginning, as opposed to striking the iron the minute you walk in the door. You haven't been there and don't really know the whole picture until you've been there for a while.

We are a family and so, with love, I want to tell you that I think that your children are not well behaved and are usually out of control.

Family and friends often feel the need to offer their opinion. (I've been on the receiving end of that!) People give an opinion about your children's behavior and activities, unsolicited.

The other thing they do that drives parents crazy is when your child is in the middle of a temper tantrum or other misbehavior, they walk up and tell you what to do. They say things like, "If you did this, instead of that, maybe they wouldn't be so upset" while you're in the middle of trying to handle it.

I would advise these people: there are a time and a place for your advice and your opinion. And the middle of a meltdown isn't the time and place.

I asked him if he needed any help. He said no, so that means everything is okay.

People often say to caregivers, "Do you need any help?" And if they say no, they assume that everything's okay. But that's usually not the case. What usually is the case is they feel uneasy about asking for help. They don't want to bother you, or they don't know what to tell you they need help with.

One of the tactics that I suggest to caregivers is to write down a list of things that you need help with, such as returning a book to a library or going to the drugstore to pick up a prescription. Then, if someone says, "Is there anything I can do to help you?" you can say, "Yes. Could you run these over to the library and pick up my books that I have on order? That would be really helpful." You're prepared.

If you're asking someone if they want your help, first, be prepared to actually help. Second, try to be specific. Say, "Is there some task or chore that I could do for you?"

When someone is caring for someone with dementia, you could make an offer along the lines of, "I can come over for two to three hours and watch reruns of *I Love Lucy* with your mom."

Another gesture that is very helpful is to send over a meal using one of the delivery services. Besides providing some relief, it makes that person feel like they're being cared about.

My son and daughter offered to help, but there's nothing they can do. They're too busy with their own lives.

I was talking to a woman who was very overwhelmed caring for her husband. I got her to tell me specifically what she could use help with. One of those things was financial management.

Her son is an accountant who lives several hours away. I asked, "Is he willing to help you?" And she said that he comes in once a month to visit her and his dad, and that he would be more than willing to help with her finances when he's in. But she said, "When he's here, I know he is tired, and I don't want to bother him."

I told her, "Let him do it. He'll feel better. He's trying to find a way to help you."

You don't realize that sometimes the person asking you actually does want to help. They want to contribute in some way. Take advantage of these offers and provide guidance for what you really need.

Solace in the Storm

Caregiving can be needed at any point in your loved ones' lives. In this book, we'll look at caregiving throughout the human lifecycle, starting with infancy. I'll also talk about how your friends and family can help, either by lending a hand or by learning what to say ... and what not to say.

Take heart; there's solace in the storm. ❧

CHAPTER 1

Caring for Young Children

Caregiving involves different responsibilities and different skills at different times in your life. As we age, so do our children, our parents, our siblings, and our spouses. And at each phase in life, our role as a caregiver can mean something new.

For many of us, the first time we take responsibility for the health and well-being of another person is when we become parents. And as parents, we face new challenges as time moves forward. Sometimes—especially with babies—the challenges seem to change daily. Other times you might have things in hand until your child's next major milestone, such as starting school or reaching puberty. Then you need to adopt a whole new set of skills.

In this chapter, I'll touch upon many of the challenges faced by parents of young children, starting with the all-consuming days of babyhood. I'll provide tips and techniques for getting through these times, and I'll also share stories from people who have been where you might be now. These stories will help you to see how to apply some of the suggestions but, more importantly, show you that, while your experience is unique to your situation, you are not alone.

A Golden Rule for Parents

Before we jump into the specific challenges that can occur throughout your child's life, if there is one lesson you take away from this chapter, it's this:

Trust your own judgment.

While you will probably lean on others to help you through difficult times—and I encourage that—when it comes down to keeping your child healthy and happy, trust your gut.

> **"**
> You know your child better than anyone else. Trust your judgment, and don't back down when you know there's an issue that needs attention.

When I worked at a community mental health center, I talked to many parents who told strikingly similar stories. Among their children, one stood out. "I knew there was something wrong with my child. I knew something was not right. I told the pediatrician, my own doctor, and my family, and everybody said, 'Don't worry about it. He'll be fine.'"

These parents knew in their heart that there was something wrong or different that needed attention. And they were almost always right.

You're the parent. You know your child better than anyone else. Trust your judgment, and don't back down when you know there's an issue that needs attention.

Feeling Overwhelmed with New Parenthood

One of the most natural feelings for a new parent is the feeling of being overwhelmed. After your baby is born, probably for the first time in your life, your time is not your own. The script for the day is determined by a tiny human who wants your attention and can ask for what they need only by crying. And their needs are constant.

People from all walks of life can become undone by this, especially if they don't have experience taking care of babies, as was the case for me. Despite my background as a child therapist, I was terrified to be left alone with a baby! Especially for CEOs and other very high-functioning professionals, the expectation is that they'll manage their new life as a parent with the same efficiency that they handle their job.

But babies do not take to being managed. They are hungry when they are hungry, not on a schedule. The result for the new parent is that simple tasks like washing the dinner dishes or folding the laundry go uncompleted. Taking a shower requires elaborate planning—if you're able to get to it at all. A trip to the grocery store is a daunting process that involves packing up the baby, keeping her entertained in the car, and finding a way to conveniently tote her while you shop. Will she start crying? Need to nurse? What used to be a simple task becomes a major project.

It's natural to feel overwhelmed simply by the logistics of your day.

Another aspect of parenting a baby that can feel overwhelming is the unsolicited input you might get from others, especially from other parents. When my oldest, Adam, was two years old, I was in a playgroup. One of the other women was a psychologist who had a little girl. She asked me, "Have you tested Adam yet?" Of course, I hadn't; he was two years old! She proceeded to tell me how high her daughter scored (on what test, I couldn't tell you!), that she was teaching her French, and that my Adam was already behind. I felt judged, inadequate as a mother, and intimidated by this woman's competitiveness and intensity. Ultimately, I had to separate myself from her.

Even my friend who was the head of a preschool—an outstanding early childhood educator—didn't find new parenthood easy. She told me about a time she was in the grocery store and her little boy kept throwing things out of the cart. She tried all her classic early childhood education techniques to get him to stop. Frustrated, exhausted, and embarrassed by the ruckus her toddler was causing, she snaked her hand up his sleeve and gave him a little pinch. The shock of it stopped him in his tracks. That trick wasn't in the parenting books (and it's not one she or I would recommend!), but it just goes to show you how tough it can be—even for a pro.

OVERWHELMED BY YOUR BABY? THESE TIPS CAN HELP!

💡 TIPS FOR THE OVERWHELMED PARENT

Ask for Help: Be specific about the timetable and your needs.

Parent in Shifts: Sleep while your partner takes a turn watching the baby, especially in the first few months.

Practice Gratitude: At a scheduled time, think of one to three things you are grateful for.

Acknowledge the Challenges: It's okay to admit you are having a rough time.

Accept Help Graciously: Set boundaries for helpers who take on more than you'd like.

You can and will get through the first years of parenthood.

First and foremost, take a moment to realize that this challenging period will not last forever. Your baby will move on to a new stage with its own challenges, but the all-consuming needs and your feeling of being out of control will pass. Hang in there!

Until then, try these techniques.

Ask for Help

This suggestion might seem obvious, but it can be the hardest to execute. Raising your hand and asking for help takes an act of will because no one wants to admit they can't do it all themselves. But if you ask, I find that family and friends are more than willing to lend a hand.

When you do ask for help, to make effective use of the time, make your request as specific as possible rather than open ended. Instead of asking for a friend or family member to come over for the afternoon to take care of your child, ask for a defined stretch of time so you can perform a specific task. For example, ask if they could come over for two hours so you can go to the grocery store or the library or so you can get outside to do some gardening. You can even ask them to watch the baby while you take a nap. When you ask people to address specific needs this way, they're much more willing to help, and you will take better advantage of the respite.

Parent in Shifts

While spending time with your partner can be the highlight of your day, when you are struggling to accomplish anything or to get some sleep, a divide-and-conquer approach is useful, at least some of the time. This is especially true when you have a colicky baby, when your child is teething and uncomfortable, or when your child is sick.

Colic presents as a period of inconsolable crying. While they used to blame colic on nervous mothers, it's actually an organic problem caused by an underdeveloped gastrointestinal system. The biggest problem with colicky babies is not just the constant crying; it's the frustration that you can't do anything about it. At the same time, you're exhausted. I've known parents with colicky babies who are trying to exist on two hours of sleep at night. It's impossible to think clearly in that state.

I knew one couple with a colicky baby, neither of whom were working at the time. The husband was a teacher and was off for the summer while the wife was on maternity leave. As loving caregivers, they were both up around the clock with the baby and were too exhausted to think of a better plan. The maternal grandmother told them, "You don't both have to be up at the same time." It didn't occur to them to care for the baby in shifts.

With a fussy and uncomfortable baby, you need someone to relieve you so you can get some sleep or rest.

For colic, it also helps to recognize that the crying has nothing to do with you and your parenting. Also, know that as the baby's GI system matures, it will stop.

Practice Gratitude

An effective technique for dealing with stress or unhappiness—whether from parenting or any other difficulties life throws at you—is to practice gratitude. Schedule some time each day—you can even set a reminder on your phone—to think of at least one thing that you are grateful for. It can be as simple as being thankful for having food on the table. Or maybe you want to think of the ways you are grateful for your partner or savor a positive moment you had with the baby. You'll be surprised by how effective this practice is at infusing your day with a dose of positivity.

Acknowledge Your Challenges

While it might seem to contradict the notion of practicing gratitude, it's also important to validate your difficult feelings. While you might not want to complain about something as precious as your new baby, it's okay to say—whether to yourself or to a patient listener—"I'm having a hard time with this." It's natural to be unhappy and frustrated. Put a name to your feelings and accept them.

Accept Help Graciously

I knew a young woman whose mother-in-law came over to help. While she was there taking care of the baby, she did some laundry and a bit of cleaning. The young woman came home and became upset. She interpreted her mother-in-law's actions as a reflection of her housekeeping as well as her parenting. But the mother-in-law thought she was being helpful, recognizing that her daughter-in-law had too much on her plate.

There are a few ways to deal with this situation. Part of it is to feel confident about asking for help. If you're not okay with it and you're not okay with someone coming into your home or taking the baby to help you, then the result will be negative for you regardless of how well it went.

Realize, too, that everybody needs help. Even people who tell you everything is fine are overwhelmed. You're not alone in needing and asking for help. So, in the case of the mother-in-law who does too much, one approach is to try not to question her motivation and learn to accept this kind of help as the blessing it is.

If you can't accept unsolicited help, communicate in advance what your needs are. "I appreciate your watching the baby. That provides so much relief. Please leave the dishes and laundry for me, though."

The more specific you are and the more you define what you really want and need, the less conflict you'll experience.

DEALING WITH NEGATIVITY

Sometimes people who think they are helping are doing the opposite. And for some people—especially other parents—boasting about their child's milestones and making you feel insecure is a way of life. What do you do about it?

When it comes to those uber-competitive parents, you have two choices: get out of the relationship or learn to laugh about it.

In my playgroup, the competitive mother made me feel so bad, I opted to leave. While I wanted to meet with other new parents, being in this group made me feel bad at a time that was already difficult for me. The bad outweighed the good.

> " You need to be around people who are positive and support you.

These decisions are difficult, but the toxicity was something I needed to remove myself from.

My leaving was based on understanding that the other mother was not going to change. Communicating to her that she was upsetting me was not going to work. That type of behavior is so ingrained, there's no stopping it. When you have very competitive parents and they're constantly comparing their child to yours, my advice is to get out of that relationship.

Sometimes you have to change your friends and avoid certain family members because of situations like this. You need to be around people who are positive and support you.

If you can learn to laugh about it, that can work, too! Someone I know referred to the competitive mom in her playgroup as "Genius Mother," and that helped her cope with the relentless bragging and comparisons.

As for the unhelpful input you get from people you can't or don't want to cut out of your life, express your needs if you can, with something like this: "I appreciate what you're saying, but I don't want to hear any more. It's not helpful."

HOW TO HELP A PARENT

⊕ QUICK TIPS: BEING A GOOD HELPER

- Offer affirmation, not solutions.
- Have a useful suggestion? Don't force it on the parents. Avoid the word "should."
- Keep greetings positive: "The baby is so sweet!" "We had fun together!"
- On the receiving end of a negativity? Write a script for how that makes you feel ... and communicate it!

You're a friend or a grandparent, and you want to help. Apart from giving your time, how do you support the new parents without making them feel judged or criticized? What do you say and not say?

First, I would encourage you to be supportive and positive. For example, I developed a therapeutic technique called *Intergenerational*

Play Therapy in which the grandparent starts each session by saying something positive about their experience with their adult child (the parent) that week. It's especially important that parents do not feel undermined when they are trying to establish their own way of doing things. Even if you don't agree with the approach, keep your feelings to yourself and be supportive unless you see a potential danger to the child.

I would also discourage the urge to swoop in and provide solutions. Instead, perhaps the most valuable thing you can do is to validate the parents' feelings. "That must be frustrating," "You sound exhausted," and "It's really hard to care for a baby" are examples of what to say. Resist the desire to relate their feelings to yours. "I know just how you feel" is not helpful. Let them own their feelings.

If you do think that something in your own experience might be helpful, it's okay to offer solutions, but be mindful of how you relay the information. You may be inclined to start off like this:

- Saying, "Why don't you ..."

- Saying, "You should ..."

- Saying something negative like, "Your child is out of control."

Instead, try sharing your experience in a nonjudgmental way.

- Start with an affirmation: "I was overwhelmed by that." "It's really difficult." "Many parents have these kinds of difficulties. You're not alone."

- Frame the advice from your point of view rather than forcing it on them: "One of the things I learned to do was ..." or "This is what I tried."

- It's especially helpful when you offer a suggestion that comes from a third party: "One of the things that someone told me to try and that worked at times was this, so I'm passing it on to you."

Taken all together, it might look like this:

"Having a colicky baby is so difficult. When Sam was fussy, someone suggested that I take him for a drive in my car. That sometimes helped. Maybe it'll help you."

How else can you improve your helper dynamics? I've been involved with many families in which the new parents asked relatives for help. The grandparents or the aunt and uncle came in to help, and when the parents came home, the first thing out of the helper's mouth was something negative: "Why weren't you doing this?" "Why didn't you do that?" "You should be doing it this way."

Criticism like this sets up a situation where the parents don't want to ask for help again. No one wants to be confronted immediately with something negative.

To be the best helper you can be, try leading with something like, "The baby and I had a really good time. What a good job you are doing!" Find something positive in the time you and the baby spent together and share it as soon as you greet the parents.

> 66
> Communicating about communicating is an art, but the more you practice, the better you'll get at it!

If you find yourself on the receiving end of a negative greeting, communicate how you feel about it. While you might feel grateful for whatever help you're getting, you can also express your needs:

"Thank you so much for your time today. I'd love to hear about how things went, but can you start with something that went right?

Then we can talk about some of the issues you noticed and what you learned that might be helpful to me."

Communicating about communicating is an art, but the more you practice, the better you'll get at it!

DEVELOPING ROUTINES THAT WORK

When it comes to parenting, I like routines. More importantly, kids like routines. It gives them structure and makes them feel secure.

One time of day that is appropriate for routines is bedtime. Setting a routine for bedtime and posting it so everybody can see it is helpful and brings structure to the home at night.

When I talk about routines to parents, they might have a bedtime or a morning routine that's not working. They might tell me that the child is difficult. But most of the time when I'm observing parents, that's not the issue.

You might also figure out who's doing each piece of the routine. Does it always have to be the same? Maybe Mom's always going to do the bedtime story because she likes to read. And maybe Dad's the one who's going to get them up and moving in the morning. Decide who's best at what and divide it up.

And then establish the routine. If you have to reevaluate it and change it, that's fine. But you have to come together as parents to decide what that routine's going to be. And then you need to try to stick to it as much as possible.

Although structure and routine are important, there needs to be some degree of flexibility in response to changes in the family's lives. Also, with older children, sometimes the routine does not work because the adults have not included the child in establishing the routine. For example, you'll find some school-aged children need a break when coming home at the end of the day before starting homework; other children want to begin imme-diately and have time for doing an activity of their choice. Each child is different. Include each of your children in establishing these routines, write it down, perhaps post it, and remind them that they agreed to this routine and they were part of the decision-making process. You will be surprised at how even young children will express what they need, when asked.

Parenting as a Unit: Don't Keep Score!

When a couple is parenting together, one issue that arises has to do with division of labor. Especially with younger couples, childcare is negotiated such that the couple ends up talking in terms of statistics: Are we sharing responsibilities 50-50, 60-40, 70-30, or something else?

But life is not a statistic, and I don't think keeping score this way is helpful. In any case, there's no standard equation that will work; the numbers change all the time as circumstances change. Drawing a line in the sand doesn't make sense logistically. Emotionally, I find it just creates conflict.

The fact is how much responsibility each partner takes on depends on work schedules, the needs of the household, and the needs of the children. Flexibility is key. What I often see is a rigid division of labor where each parent might do the routine on set nights of the week. And often there's no flexibility to say that maybe you're not up to it and you want the other partner to step up even though it's not "their night." What ends up happening is the parents end up fighting about it. Being flexible is important for these routines to work.

To make parenting together work, one approach is to make up a schedule each week that's based on everyone's work and other commitments and the children's needs. Pick a night that works for you for working out the schedule for the week; using a whiteboard can be helpful. Then work out the details: Your child needs to be picked up from day care Monday night and Dad is done with work early, so he's going to do it that night. Maybe he'll also do pickup on Tuesday because Mom is going to yoga that night. But on Wednesday he has a late dinner meeting and Mom is done early, so now Mom is going to pick up the child.

What you don't want to do when coming up with this schedule is to add up how many hours one parent is spending versus the other parent. The goal is to find something that works for everyone in your family, not to balance out the numbers.

Dads as Caregivers

Today, it's very common to see men taking care of kids. It's becoming more culturally acceptable, and men feel increasingly comfortable in the role. While times are changing and seeing dads as equal or even primary caregivers is not uncommon, I still find dads in these roles who are either being given a hard time or, as primary caregivers, struggling with isolation.

DEALING WITH FAMILY OPINIONS

Some family members—often the grandparents—are stuck in a traditional way of thinking. I remember when I was raising my children. My husband was as involved as he could be, given his hectic work schedule. My mother-in-law was at our house one day, and witnessing my husband's hands-on approach, she clucked with disapproval. "His father would *never* have done that."

That wasn't helpful. Supportive grandparents make things easier; the opposite is also true.

Grandparents need to accept that today, with both parents working (or just because he wants to), fathers are going to, at a minimum, pitch in. It's good for the children to have both parents as caregivers. It takes some of the load off the mother, and it gives the children a different perspective of life. Not to be supportive of a father being a caregiver takes that away from the children.

As for extended family, I often see issues arise during family events. A baby starts crying or a toddler throws a tantrum, and the father gets up to handle it. There might be negative comments made and jokes that are not positive. I advise family members that they need to be supportive of this man helping his partner. The better response than sarcasm or joking at the father's expense is to be positive. "That's so great that you got up from dinner to pick up the baby."

How do you, as a parent, make that happen? I like scripts for this purpose. Preparing what you are going to say ahead of time makes you more confident when you share your thoughts. So, sometimes I tell young men and women to develop a script for this situation (and deliver it) something like this:

> *What you're saying is not acceptable. What you can say is [whatever you'd like them to say], which would be helpful. What you're saying creates problems and conflict. It's becoming such a problem that it's uncomfortable for us, and we don't look forward to coming for dinner. Here are the choices: do not make any comments, or say [something positive], and then we will continue to enjoy each other.*

Give them the words you want them to say because they are not going to figure it out themselves.

BEING APPRECIATIVE

I often find that moms tend to see dads helping with the care as just part of their responsibility. So why should they get praised for that?

Everyone likes praise. Moms need to recognize that fathers as caregivers need as much support and recognition as they want and deserve as mothers. I've seen situations where, on Mother's Day, there's a lot of hoopla and flowers and gifts, and the kids making breakfast in bed for Mom. Then, when Father's Day comes along, the celebration is much more subdued. But I would encourage the same level of celebration for Dad as there is for Mom and to otherwise be generous with praise.

THE STAY-AT-HOME DAD

In a household where the family decides the dad will stay home to care for the children, I see a few issues. One is that the men run into a lot of prejudice. People might judge the dad's ability to make a living or make assumptions about the family's finances.

I knew one dad who, when he would go into a doctor's office, a nurse would ask, "Where's the mom?" And he would have to speak up, "I'm here. I'm a parent, and I'm here."

When it comes to friends and acquaintances, you don't need to explain or justify your decision. Whether the decision is financial or logistical, it's none of anyone's business. Stick to the main point: this is what we decided for our family.

To deal with the pushback you might get from your relatives, being subtle about your decision or letting them make inferences won't work. Be up front about it. Tell them, "This is what we've decided as a couple. This is how we're going to raise our family. We feel very comfortable with this."

If they start to voice opinions, bring out your boundaries. I find that when you are clear about your intentions and you're both saying the same thing, people accept it.

The other thing I hear stay-at-home dads complain about is feeling isolated. They take their children to the playground or the library and mostly women are there. Some men are able to build friendships with women in these settings. Many find the dynamic doesn't work.

What I suggest for these men is to try to find other men who are caregivers. One way to do this is to go to your house of worship or some other organization in your community to see if they run a parenting group in which men are active or if they will form one. It might take a little effort to find one or get one started, but once you're involved in this kind of group, it can be very helpful.

Over time, you might not stay in the group because you don't need the formal group as much as you need the relationships. Once you have those relationships, you'll begin to get together with the children, find shared interests and activities, and feel less alone.

On Their Best Behavior

How do you get your children to do what you want? Perhaps more importantly, how do you prevent or stop them from doing what you don't want? Getting your children to behave is one of the biggest challenges of parenting young children. Let's look at some behavior issues you are apt to encounter—from tantrums to lying—and what you can do about them.

THOSE TERRIBLE TANTRUMS!

Kids are very good at figuring out that, if they throw a tantrum in a public place, you will probably give in to them to avoid embarrassment. This is especially hard if you regard your child's behavior as a direct reflection of you. If you do, you will immediately capitulate to their demands.

But understand that all children have behavior issues at times, and that's not necessarily a reflection of you as a parent. If you can separate your feelings from their behavior, dealing with tantrums becomes a little easier.

When that tantrum does come, what do you do? When a child has a temper tantrum in a public place, the hardest thing to do is to remove them from the situation, but sometimes you have to. I have picked up my children and carried them out, even if it meant leaving a half-full grocery cart in the middle of the cereal aisle.

You can also try putting them in quiet time with you in an unbusy area of the store. Whatever you do, you can't give into the tantrums. Because they're only going to get worse.

It also helps to know that a tantrum usually comes in stages. It escalates and then ends as a temper tantrum. Try to become aware of your child's stages before they get to that full-blown temper tantrum, and try to intervene at a much earlier point. Sometimes I see children and it's obvious to me on the outside looking in that they're very tired or they're very hot or they've just had it. And they're building, they're getting there.

The parent, who's also probably tired and hot, needed to try to intervene at an earlier point and say, "This isn't going to work today." Because in five minutes they're going to have a full-blown tantrum.

What if your child tends to tantrum every time you do a particular activity? For example, suppose you visit a friend at their house or out for coffee on a regular basis. Every time you go, your child melts down when you try to get them out of the car.

Depending on the age of the child, you might ask them what their issue is. Maybe the friend has a child your child doesn't like to play with. Maybe they're bored. Then the question becomes, "What can we do during that time to occupy you?" And maybe you're going to give them a video game for an hour. Sometimes you need to break the rules.

So don't forget to ask questions. They know why they're having a fit. Ask, "What's going on?" Usually, they will tell you, and then you can at least attempt to address the problem.

What's less effective is to give a long speech. Explaining endlessly usually doesn't help. Understand the root of the problem, and then try to address it.

And sometimes, you just have to take action! I remember leaving my son with my parents for the first time, and he was upset. I spent a lot of time explaining to him why it was okay and that he would be all right. My father overheard and said, "It's enough already! Stop talking! Leave!" He was right. Sometimes we don't need these long conversations. Just do what you need to do. By the way, my father later told me that once we left, our son calmed down and had a great time with his grandparents.

DISCIPLINING CHILDREN

While disciplining children can be a vast topic, I generally advocate a three-step process. Unfortunately, the third step is rarely taken, which leads to ongoing problems.

The first step is to interrupt the behavior. Suppose your child is jumping on the furniture and making a lot of noise. Stop them so that you can have a conversation about it.

The second step is to identify to the child what they're doing that they shouldn't be doing. "I've asked you not to jump on the furniture like that. Please don't do that."

And that's usually where the discipline stops. But you need to go further!

The third step—the one that is often forgotten about—is to teach a new behavior. They don't always know how to stop what they are doing. Maybe the child has excess energy they need to burn off. So, for example, you can put on some music and suggest they move to the rhythm instead.

The message to them is "You don't need to do that. When you run into this situation, here are some things you can do instead."

WHEN A CHILD HITS

When a child is angry and hits another person, saying to a child, "Use your words" won't help them to get rid of the anger. They need a combination of words and some physical action that doesn't hurt anyone to express their anger. When a child is really angry, using just words is not a complete solution for someone who's young and immature. Find an alternative way for them to express their anger. Your child might even have their own ideas for how to do that. And eventually, they will transition to using their words.

MODIFYING BEHAVIOR THROUGH PLAY

MAKING THE MOST OF PLAYTIME WITH YOUR CHILD

When you're playing games and doing other activities with your children, *listen*. Playing together is an opportunity to learn how your child thinks and how they're feeling. When they're engrossed in a game, they're talking. And what they're talking about and how they're reacting to the game gives you an opportunity as a parent to learn more about your child, not just their thoughts and feelings but how they react to certain situations, such as losing.

Learning to lose is a skill, and how your child reacts to losing can be an opportunity for you to have a conversation about it. Whatever the game, playing together gives you many opportunities to communicate and interact with your child.

I often teach parents to use play as a reward for their child performing a desired behavior. You can use activities such as playing with your child or reading to your child to modify their behavior.

The approach is to tell your child that if they do whatever it is you want them to do for the time you specify, you will spend a certain amount of time doing the reward activity. You can use this technique for any behavior you are looking for, from doing a chore to doing homework, to being quiet so you can complete a task.

The offer might look like, "If you spend twenty minutes quietly doing your homework, I will spend ten minutes playing your favorite game with you."

Don't worry about how much time you spend with them. It doesn't have to be an hour or an afternoon (although it can be if that makes sense to you).

When you use this technique, it's important to set a timer. Also, understand that your end of the bargain is to put your phone away during your time together. Your full attention must be paid to your child. When the timer goes off, you can go back to doing whatever you were doing. But for the promised minutes, you need to be fully engaged with your child.

This technique is highly effective, and you will likely find that you can relax and enjoy it. It's good for you as well as for the child, and the child learns that, if they want that attention, they can do what they need to do to get undivided time.

In terms of the activity you perform, you can let your child lead the way. You can also think about what you liked to do as a kid. What was your favorite play activity? Whether it's coloring books or puzzles or LEGOs, that can be a good place to start. What's really important to the child is their time with you, not what they're doing. While there's a theory that you always have to follow the child's lead, when you're first starting to spend time with your child this way, sometimes it's easier to start with something you enjoy doing.

What if they want to do an activity that you really don't enjoy? You can offer to do their activity for, say, ten minutes, but then you're going to do something different. Negotiation is fine: we'll play your game, and then let's play mine.

WHEN CHILDREN LIE

Lying is a normal developmental stage that typically occurs between the ages of six to eight. While you can't allow it, understand the reason it's happening is that the child has developed cognitively, and they suddenly realize that you, as their parent, do not actually possess knowledge of what is always going on in the universe. They realize that you don't have eyes in the back of your head, and you don't know what's going on at all times in every place.

If you recognize why children lie, then sometimes understanding the issue from their perspective makes it easier to solve the issue. Some of the main reasons why children lie are as follows:

- To avoid punishment. This applies to any age, from breaking an object in the house to violating a curfew or lying about where they were and who they were with.

- To gain an advantage. Examples include cheating on a test or telling a false tale to another child about someone else to get them to like them better than the other person.

- To remove themselves from an uncomfortable situation. For example, they know that someone was not invited to a party, and so they tell them that they weren't invited either.

How do you deal with lying? It's a matter of having consequences and making them very clear. "If you're lying, I will find out. And if I catch you in a lie, here are the consequences for that."

When you're giving consequences to children, have them repeat the condition and the consequence to you because you want to make sure they understand it.

> 66
> When you're giving consequences to children, have them repeat the condition and the consequence to you because you want to make sure they understand it.

This same developmental phase might result in other forms of misbehavior, such as suddenly not following rules. It's the same issue. They come to realize they have power, and they don't necessarily have to follow the rules; they can go their own way. They are testing the boundaries. Again, realize it's developmentally appropriate. At the same time, deal with the behavior firmly when you do encounter it.

 QUICK TIPS: HOMEWORK

I don't like sending kids—especially young kids—to their room to do homework. It can be too distracting. It's more effective to have everybody sitting at the table together. It doesn't matter what *you* do during that time; just be there and be available in case someone needs help. And if your child does become distracted, you're there to help them to refocus on their work.

KEEPING TECHNOLOGY IN ITS PLACE

More and more, technology is a part of young children's lives. There are lots of resources and software programs that allow you to control how much time your child is spending online that you can find by searching the internet. Some software allows you to see what they're doing. I've had discussions with a few parents who think that's invading their child's privacy by doing so. When your child is ten years old, it's okay to monitor their activity.

One thing about technology that parents lose sight of is that, like everything else, you have to model the appropriate behavior. If you're sitting down to dinner and you are on your phone, don't be surprised when your children end up doing the same.

For parents, the help you find on the internet can be a godsend. But there's an old story in which a baby is crying. The parents are standing by the crib and they're flipping through a childcare book trying to figure out what's going on. And the grandmother walks in, looks at the parents, and says, "Put down the book, pick up the baby."

Now I say, "Put down the phone and pick up your child or look at your child." I've seen parents stand in the shallow end of a pool supposedly watching their children while they are constantly on their phone. The allure of the phone can be powerful, but don't let it come between you and your child.

Rituals

Rituals create memories that bind a family together. I've found that especially to be the case with children who are adopted. If you're adopting a child who's a little older, when they you bring them home, you can have balloons, a cake, a celebratory dinner, and so on.

You can create a ceremony and a ritual for the day that they came into the family, assuming the child is all right with that. Most children are okay with it. They celebrate their birthday, and then they also celebrate the day they became part of your family. It's a way of binding the family together and also saying, "This is important. And this is how we celebrate it."

When You Know Something Isn't Right

A five-year-old child was referred to me by a day care center. They thought the child had serious mental health issues. I met the child, along with her mother and grandmother, and she was talking about things that were a little off. She didn't sound psychotic—just a little strange. Listening to her was almost like listening to a soap opera. But when I asked the mother if the child watched any daytime TV, she assured me she didn't.

While working with the child using a therapeutic game, I discovered that she was not only reading but that she was an advanced reader for her age. Through more questioning, I learned that she had been secretly reading her grandmother's romance novels. That explained the odd dialogue!

I talked with the teacher and explained that the child could read and suggested they move her to the gifted program. But the teacher said, "My recommendation will be that she go to the behavioral classroom."

But then I tested the child, and she tested very high. Her behavior issues in class were likely related to being bored. She belonged in the gifted program.

The mother didn't know how to handle the situation. The teacher was telling her that her daughter belonged in the behavioral room. The mom felt powerless to disagree and was having difficulty speaking up. She viewed the teacher as the authority.

I ended up writing a script for her that would oblige the school to test her. The language to use has to do with accommodating your child. As a parent, you have to tell the principal that your child has special needs and is not being accommodated. Then you tell them that you are requesting testing to be done by the school psychologist in order to define and meet these needs.

After the school tested the child, as expected she scored extremely high, and they ended up putting her in the gifted program, as I had suggested. But if I hadn't given the words to the mom—who was a wonderful mother—she might have gone along with what the teacher said, even though in her heart she knew it was the wrong solution.

Situations like this can happen with a behavior, educational, or health issue. Professionals are telling you one thing, but you know they are not right. What do you do?

Here are a few practices that are effective:

- Consult your own professional.

- If you don't agree with that professional, get a second opinion.

- Need a specialist? You can google specialists, search the directory on your local hospital's website, and ask friends and others in your personal network. You can also ask your doctor for a referral.

- Insist that the school test your child to find out what's really going on.

For learning issues, you can request or, if necessary, demand a parent-teacher conference that involves more than the teacher. You can involve the principal and the educational specialists in the school. You can also bring your family's psychologist or counselor into those meetings so that you have more people who support you. These professionals also know how to get the school to take actions that they might refuse if only you were asking.

You might also want to get your own neuropsychological exam for your child, in addition to the school's testing. That can be challenging. A neuropsych exam can run between $2,000 and $3,000. This might not be covered by insurance, so discuss this with your child's pediatrician or counselor, with your insurance company, and with other parents to learn about the strategies you can use to get coverage.

There are also educational specialists that work privately. You will need to pay out of pocket for this option, but these specialists have a lot of experience dealing with special education and might be able to help you when others can't.

Learning to Lose / Accepting Failure

The term "helicopter parent" is an apt description for parents who hover around their children, shielding them from any negative experience or intervening on their behalf. It might feel like you are protecting them from heartache, but when a child isn't allowed to recognize that they made a mistake or to lose, they never learn the skills of working through these experiences. They need to learn how to accept failure and how to recover. They have to learn to trust themselves. They should be able to say to themselves, "I have failed before and survived, and I know I'm going to get through it again this time."

If they don't have this experience as children, they end up as adults who fall apart at the first failure that they have to handle on their own. I've seen people go into deep depressions; they start drinking or abusing other substances. They can't handle adversity because they have no coping skills.

Your job as a parent is to help them accept the loss. Say to them: You got a bad grade on a test? Yes, that happened. Let's talk about what you're going to do so that doesn't happen again. You lost a Little League game? Yes, you did. You're not going to win every game, let's just get through it. I've seen parents cover it up; they don't allow the child to experience the loss.

One of my sons played football. After a loss, my tactic was to say, "Let's settle down. Think through what happened and what you can do differently the next time, or what you can, as a team, do differently the next time. Sometimes the reality is the other team was just better. Sometimes the other team was stronger. And you can get stronger and better, but you have to work on it. And even if you do, you won't win every game."

TAKEAWAY: "SMOOTH WATERS DO NOT MAKE FOR GOOD SAILORS"

This African proverb is a favorite quote of mine. The fact is that all of us wish for smooth seas for our children, but we know that the waters are never smooth. A feeling of competency and trust in oneself is a result of having ridden out the storm successfully. If you have never experienced a storm or rough waters or someone else has always piloted the boat, then you lack faith in your ability to succeed. An individual's self-esteem can crumble quickly when suddenly faced with heavy seas. Thus, the ability to experience failure, and from that failure, to go on to succeed is a gift. It grants a sense of inner pride in our own competency and ability to manage the boat through the sea of life.

Children Grow …

And before you know it, they've reached adolescence! I'll talk about the issues you'll face during these years in the next chapter. ❧

CHAPTER 2

Caring for Adolescent Children

While the time between your child's birth and puberty comes with an ever-changing set of challenges, adolescence can bring a dramatic turnabout in your child's behavior. It's a turbulent and confusing time not just for teenagers but for their parents. Adolescents are experiencing body changes, oftentimes mood swings that are beyond their control, and stress from school, athletics, family members, and peers. They could be a victim of bullying or experience an eating disorder, substance abuse, alcoholism, or sexual pressures, just to name a few of the problems that can arise.

A Helpful Foundation

One of the important changes that occurs in adolescence that differentiates it somewhat from early childhood is that many of the variables that impact adolescence are interrelated. One issue might produce problems in multiple areas. To discuss responses and possible remedies in only one domain at a time is limiting. So before we look at some of the problems you might come up against during the adolescent years, I'd like to start this chapter by sharing with you some general guidelines that will help you across the board.

💡 QUICK TIPS TO CARING FOR ADOLESCENTS

- Establish good communication practices before your children become teens.
- Avoid being judgmental.
- Encourage solutions that fit your child's personality and temperament.
- Discuss adolescence with your child before its onset.
- Propose an alternative adult to talk to if talking to you about certain issues is difficult for them.
- Accept that they are trying to figure out who they are. Let them find themselves.
- Help your teen to establish healthy patterns around sleeping and eating.
- Model nonviolent behavior.
- Volunteer in your child's school as much as possible.
- Teach them important life skills, like time management.

Start having open and calm discussions with your child before they become teenagers. Building a foundation of trust and openness will help you to communicate with your teenager when the seas become rough.

Practice nonjudgmental communication. Although it is very difficult, listen instead of lecturing. Try not to offer too much advice too quickly.

Encourage your child to find solutions that match their personal style and with which they feel comfortable. Teaching them how to analyze situations and find solutions is a skill they will use throughout their life.

If they are not comfortable discussing certain issues with you, consider having your child speak with a trusted friend or family

> 66
> **Adolescents are trying to define who they are.** Rebellion and disagreement are among the ways in which they discover who they are and who they want to be.

member. Sometimes your child might feel more comfortable talking with an adult other than you, like a grandparent. Some situations might even require the services of a professional such as a physician or a psychologist.

Prepare for changes in advance. Before your child hits puberty, talk about changes that might be on the horizon for them.

- Changes in their bodies.

- Changes in their feelings or moods.

- Pressure from peers, teachers, or coaches.

This approach can help your child to be better prepared. Share your own experiences. Your child may look disinterested, but if they are in the room, they are listening.

Adolescents are trying to define who they are. Rebellion and disagreement are among the ways in which they discover who they are and who they want to be.

I once had an adolescent patient who was arguing with his parents about religion. The parents were not religious and had decided to allow their children to explore all possibilities and choose the religion they wanted—if any. In the session, the boy kept demanding to know his parents' religions. They kept trying to stay neutral by not naming the religions in which they were raised. The father was getting very frustrated and finally screamed, "Why is it so important for you to know what religion I am?" His son replied, "So that I can make sure that I choose differently."

On the surface this appeared to be a child who was being difficult, but he really was trying to define himself as an individual. This is difficult to live with but an important part of the growth process.

BEING PRESENT

I found one of the most effective ways to communicate with my children was to hang out in their bedrooms or the living room and not say a word. When you are in the vicinity and are completely silent, individuals, even your children, will begin to talk to you. *Just listen.* The most important thing you can do when they begin to talk to you is to keep your mouth shut. Do not offer opinions or advice. Be engaged and listen intently. You will learn a lot.

If you feel the need to comment you can always do so later.

Routines and expected behaviors with defined consequences provide boundaries and stability for adolescents who are suffering numerous anxieties. Sleep, healthy eating, and exercise are important elements for controlling stress. Dr. Michael Breus, an author, psychologist, and sleep expert, has written about how sleeping patterns change depending on the age of the child. A normal sleeping pattern for most teens is to sleep later and stay up later.[2]

Healthy eating and exercise begin with you as a parent. Assess the food that is available in your home, your own eating patterns, and exercise routines, and consider how you can model the behavior you expect from your teen.

Try to be flexible with routines and behavioral expectations. Chores and responsibilities in the home are important. However, you might consider excusing your teen from some of these expectations during exam periods such as midterms and finals.

When I was a young adult, I was responsible for working with the bookkeeper in my father's business by preparing the books for the accountant at the end of every month. I was always relieved when my college exams fell at the end of the month, as I was excused from these responsibilities.

Violence begets violent behavior. If your child has been disciplined in a violent manner or has observed violence in your home, then in times of stress, they will revert to a pattern of verbal or physically aggressive behavior.

Volunteer. I found the easiest way to stay "in-the-know" about how a teen is doing in school and their relationships with teachers and friends is to volunteer as much as possible in their school. This might be challenging depending on your work schedule but try to be there as much as possible.

Teach your teen important life skills. Essential skills include being assertive, budgeting their time (including how to manage both

---

2   Dr. Michael Breus, "Teens Need More Sleep than You Think," The Sleep Doctor, published on May 19, 2022, https://thesleepdoctor.com/author/dr-michael-breus/.

short- and long-term projects), learning how to set realistic expectations, and problem solving.

💡 QUICK TIP: EXPERIENCE THEIR WORLD

If you want to learn more about how your child is thinking, what their values are, and how they view the world, then enter their world. Read the same books they do and then discuss the characters. Watch the same television shows and movies. Read their fan fiction—whatever is the portal into their world. Doing so will give you a common set of experiences and a common language.

With these guidelines as a basis and recognizing that solutions are not always simple and clear-cut, I'd like to offer some insight into some of the issues you might encounter as your child progresses through adolescence.

Their Changing Bodies and Demeanors

I have a friend whose oldest daughter had always been a kind and a happy child. Whenever I visited and she came home from school, she would say hello to me, kiss her mother, and sit for a few minutes to chat with us.

One day when I was visiting, she came through the door, and we said hello. She abruptly turned away, ran up the stairs, and slammed her bedroom door. When I asked my friend if she was going upstairs to see what the matter was, she calmly replied, "Welcome to fourteen years old and hormones!"

My friend assured me that she spoke to her daughter often and knew what was going on in her life. However, there were times when her daughter needed to be alone with her feelings. The upshot is to be there for them when they need to talk or are ready to talk. But also give them the space to be a teen and work through their emotions on their own.

Keeping Technology in Check

Herein lies the golden rule: the behavior you model is the behavior that your children will follow.

You can install all the fancy software you want that shuts off their phones and computers at a specific time. I recommend this practice; it imposes a limit on their use of technology and forces them to go to sleep and do their homework and chores and so on. (You can also simply take away the phone at key times, such as just before bedtime.) However, children often figure out how to get around policing software and apps.

If you lecture them about the overuse of technology and yet you are sitting at dinner and are constantly on the phone, that communicates a different behavior. Use restraint with regard to your own phone if you expect your children to do the same.

☀ QUICK TIP: CAR TIME

You'll be surprised by what you learn from your teen if you let the quiet of the car work for you.

While you won't be fiddling with your phone while you are driving for safety reasons, you might be tempted to use car time to talk on the phone hands free to catch up on conversations with friends and business associates. While your adolescent is in the car, though, I suggest refraining from phone conversations as much as possible. The car is an excellent place for spontaneous conversations with your teen. Because you are not making eye contact, it can be easier to talk about random topics. This type of conversation both gives you information you might not otherwise get and also can help to bring you closer.

This holds true even when their friends are in the car—*especially* when their friends are in the car. You can be a fly on the wall or, if you're invited, a participant in the conversation. You will learn a lot about what they are talking about and what's important to them at the moment.

Bullying

Very much related to the issue of technology is bullying. These days, a lot of bullying occurs on social media or over text. And because of the use of technology, it's hard to stop it.

But the main problem is that parents often don't know that it's happening. Kids don't want to disclose bullying incidents to their parents because they're embarrassed and ashamed or because they don't want to be seen as a tattletale. That can get them into bad situations. Some bullied children become suicidal, and some do go on to commit suicide.

That brings us back to the issue of open communication and creating an environment in which your child feels that they can come to you.

It's also a good idea for them to have alternate pathways for communication that you identify and say are okay. You can tell your child,

"If you don't feel comfortable talking to me, that's okay. You can talk to your grandfather, or you could talk to your Uncle John. Those are people you could go to, to confide in. And I'm okay with that." And then you need to really be okay with that because they have to have these pathways when something is going on.

If you do find out that your child is being bullied, you need to notify the school. It might make things difficult for your child, but they're going to have to try to live through what happens with kids at school when they say something because it has to be reported.

The other thing I would do with my bullied child is have them shut down all their online communications for the moment. Cancel social media accounts; get a new phone number. Explain to them that the purpose of bullying is to upset you. Explain to them that if you're not responding to it and you ask your friends not to respond to it, so you've basically shut them down and blocked them, then they've lost their pathway to you. They're going to move on to somebody else.

As a parent, you need to address bullying as if someone were literally holding a weapon because it *is* a weapon, and it's very, very dangerous. While shutting down their social media presence can be hard, they can then open up a new technical means of communication that only one or two of their very best and trusted friends have.

Because it's so important to keep your child safe, another alternative—probably the last resort—is to remove them from their current school. Depending on where you live, there might be alternatives like charter schools, but I've found that usually if you tell the school system you want to move them and the reason why, they're pretty responsive to that.

I've known parents who have taken a change in the school system as an opportunity. One parent I was speaking to recently has a child who is very involved with theater. She was having huge problems in the school she was at. They moved her to another school where theater arts was basically a minor for her. And she's done very, very well there. She sings and participates in the theater arts division. The kids like her. For the first time in her life, she really has friends. Parents, when thinking about moving a child to another school, ought to see it as an opportunity to perhaps make a positive change in the child's curriculum or extracurricular activities

The other thing I've had parents do, when it's possible and they want to, is move into homeschooling for a while. I've known parents who can't do the homeschooling themselves but have hired tutors to come in to teach, which is an option if you can afford that. But know that getting your child out of the school system can cool things down such that the bullies move on.

Discipline in the Teen Years

We discussed in chapter 1 the three steps in the disciplinary process, which apply at any age.

- Interrupt the behavior.

- Identify what they're doing that they shouldn't be doing.

- Teach a new behavior.

However, for adolescents it's especially important to have clear consequences for refusing to follow the rules. Here are some guidelines for consequences.

MAKE CONSEQUENCES AGE APPROPRIATE AND ENFORCEABLE

Make sure that any consequence is age appropriate and that you will be able to enforce it. For example, if you are planning on going to a special event that you really want to attend, don't use it as a consequence unless you are willing to forgo the event and stay at home with your child. If missing the event is the consequence, who's being punished?

CONSEQUENCES SHOULD BE CLEAR AND NONNEGOTIABLE

When my sons began driving, we established the rules concerning curfews and the consequences. The rule was that if they were late and had not called to inform us that they were going to be late and ask for permission to be late, then they would lose their car for one week. We would not yell at them, but if they violated their curfew, we would simply be standing at the front door as they entered, with a hand out to collect their car keys. No arguing and no negotiating; just hand over the keys to your car.

Herb Cohen, an American negotiation expert and author of several books on the topic, wrote that business negotiations were often like those with adolescents. They ask for something, and you clearly say no. Do they stop there? No. They consider your response the beginning of the negotiation. The lesson? Don't get sucked in to too much discussion and negotiation. Keep it simple: here is the rule; here is the consequence. End of discussion.

PICK YOUR BATTLES

Not everything your adolescent does that you don't like requires inter-vention and consequences. When our youngest son wanted a rattail (a long, thin ponytail), my husband became very upset. I told him to let it go. Our son played football, and I knew that the first time a player on the opposing team grabbed him by that tail, that would be the end of it. And that's exactly what happened; an opponent used it as a handle to pull him down. The rattail was gone the next day.

> So don't make a big deal out of every disagreement.

So don't make a big deal out of every disagreement. Often these things have a way of taking care of themselves.

ACCEPTING THE CONSEQUENCES

Some parents protect their child no matter what they do and try to get them to avoid consequences. If you're overly invested in your child as an athlete or as a student vying for a scholarship to an Ivy League school, then you might help them to avoid consequences for misbehavior or poor performance.

We talked in chapter 1 about how it's important to allow your child to fail so they develop resilience. But this issue also reflects on how ego involved you are in your child's success. Realize, too, that you're setting a pattern for how the child is going to continue to operate for the rest of their life.

Consider the recent "Varsity Blues" case in which wealthy parents—including some celebrities—paid off coaches and the like to manipulate the college admissions process. Maybe the student goofed off, never went to class, and wasn't a good student. When the parent intervenes, that child is going to expect an easy ride for the rest of their life. They're going to feel as though they don't have to produce or don't have to work because they can pay off somebody to get what they want.

Another way in which parents sometimes run interference is when a teacher calls and says, "There's an issue here." Does the parent address the issue with the child? Often, the parent instead blames it on the teacher. When that happens, you need to decide. Are you going to raise the child to become a responsible adult member of a community? Are you going to hold them responsible for their actions? That's really the decision point, and parents have to think that through. Making your child accept the consequences can be very, very difficult, but you're setting up a foundation for a lifetime.

Of course, there are situations in which the teacher or coach or other adult in a position of authority is wrong. I've had kids in treatment where I absolutely did not agree with the teacher, and I think the teacher was wrong. But in other situations—probably most situations—the teacher was very right and there needed to be consequences to the child.

High-Risk Behaviors

The adolescent years can be a minefield. Perhaps you remember your own teen years and some of the risky behaviors you were exposed to. How, you may wonder, can you protect your adolescent during this time that is fraught with opportunity for them to hurt themselves?

BUILDING TRUST WITH YOUR CHILD

While you won't want to abdicate your responsibility as a parent and become your child's pal, you will probably want to create a more open and less judgmental rapport with them than you likely had with your own parents. You want them to feel comfortable coming to you when something important is on their mind. How do you do this? Here are a few ideas:

- Be supportive of who they are, not of who you want them to be.

- Don't be overly critical.

- While consequences are important, don't yell and create a fear-based relationship.

- Teach them how to solve problems.

Probably the best tool you have is keeping the lines of communication open. Regardless of your relationship with your child, though, problems can arise.

DRUG ABUSE

One of the ways that drug abuse happens these days is at what's called a *pharma party*. The teens walk into the party and there's a large goblet or bowl. Everyone throws in pills that they've taken from their home. Then they pick a pill or two at random and take them.

It's practices like this that make your bathroom the highest-risk room in your house. Your children and their friends have access to anything they want in there, as the bathroom is the one place that they are not supervised.

Because of these parties and other situations, one tip is to make sure you safely dispose of any unnecessary medications in your medicine cabinets. You might have been given a painkiller for a procedure and took only one or two pills. That bottle is still in your bathroom. Dispose of it. But don't flush the medications down the toilet. You can generally dispose of medications at your local pharmacy or at a police station.

Also be aware that ADHD medications are very popular targets for abuse among adolescents. If your child is prescribed medications like Adderall or Ritalin, be attentive to whether they are taking them and not sharing them with their friends.

DRUNK DRIVING / RIDING WITH A DRUNK FRIEND

THE DRUNK DRIVING PROBLEM

According to the Centers for Disease Control (CDC), while teen drunk driving has lessened over the last thirty years, high school teens drive after drinking about 2.4 million times a month.[3]

It's important to give your children alternatives to getting behind the wheel or getting in the passenger seat when alcohol is involved. One approach is to give your child what I used to call an emergency credit card, which means they can use the credit card when they're in an emergency situation and need to get home safely. They can call a taxi or an Uber if they don't want to call you.

---

3   "Teen Drinking and Driving," cdc.gov (Centers for Disease Control and Prevention, October 2012), https://www.cdc.gov/vitalsigns/teendrinkinganddriving/index.html.

The big, important thing is to tell them that there will be no questions asked if they do make one of those calls. Because if they think you're going to drill them, they won't call you or use your credit card. They'll get in the car with the person who's driving, even if they're drunk.

The other thing I did with my kids was to tell them that they could call one of the other moms in the neighborhood if they felt uncomfortable calling me. We had four or five moms who all lived in the same neighborhood. We had an unwritten agreement between us that we would tell our kids to call one of the moms and that any help they asked for would be kept confidential. The important thing was keeping them safe, not to catch them getting into trouble.

This pact extended beyond the drunk driving situation. If we saw something happening with a child that we thought wasn't safe, we agreed to interfere and try to stop them. Or if one of the kids needed something or wanted something, they could call any one of us in this group of moms.

It's helpful to form those alliances and that you commit to helping each other out. I have a friend who's Argentinian. She was in Argentina visiting her family. I got a call at two o'clock in the morning. Her son was in the emergency room. She asked me, "Merle, can you get to the emergency room? I'm scared to death. I don't know what's going on. He's in there, and can you get there?"

And I went. She would've done the same thing for me because we had this understanding that we were going to help each other out. If you haven't already, work to build these types of relationships and establish agreements with each other.

Your Adolescent's Health

Two of the biggest issues with regard to your child's health concern weight and being sexually active.

OBESITY

Obesity is a huge problem in this country. It's caused both by bad eating habits and lack of exercise. In terms of the eating habits, there are three big issues.

- Your own eating and modeling good eating habits.

- The foods you have available in the house.

- Dependence on fast foods.

If you keep unhealthy snacks and junk food in the house, and you're constantly having arguments about how many cookies or treats your child can have, you can either argue about it or just keep the treats out of the house if your kid is overweight. It's a hard problem.

The other hard problem is type 1 diabetes, which is on the rise in young people. The child might have a predisposition to it, overload on sugar, and trigger the disease. We discussed this on my podcast, and the feeling from the endocrinologist that I had on was—and he's done a lot of research in this area—the availability of fast food. His research showed there was a correlation between a jump in type 1 diabetes and the number of fast-food restaurants in the local area.

If you do have a child who has type 1 diabetes, the issue eventually becomes how do they live their life as a teenager when all of their friends are out eating pizza and other foods they aren't allowed? They've got to watch their diet, and it's really difficult for them. There have been books written now on helping your adolescent or your college student deal with type 1 diabetes because eating is a social activity, and it becomes a huge problem for them.

ANOREXIA

Anorexia often is blamed on the American culture, but that's not exactly accurate. Everyone thinks it has to do with the American culture and that the aesthetic ideal of these very, very thin people. And so teenage girls are trying to get to that. But the research really doesn't support that.

It's really the good girl, bad girl problem. And in order to be a good girl, you have to look a certain way, and you have to do all these other things that way. And that's really what is behind the psychodynamics in anorexia.

SEXUAL ACTIVITY AND PREGNANCY

Another health issue has to do with being sexually active, preventing pregnancy, and sexually transmitted diseases.

Once again, I can't stress enough the importance of keeping the doors of communication open. If you're comfortable talking about it, then your adolescents will talk to you about it. If they've been raised in a judgmental and punitive environment, they are less likely to talk to you. And it can be important for them to talk to you so they can ask you to bring them to a physician to assist them in making safe decisions.

I was pretty blunt with my boys. I wasn't going to get into a discussion of whether or not they should be sexually active. When my boys were growing up it was the age of AIDS and sexually transmitted diseases, which is what I was most concerned about.

I told them that unprotected sex wasn't a mistake where you can say, "Oops! I made a mistake; I won't do that again." Because if you get the disease, or you've made someone pregnant, it's a problem you cannot easily correct for. And I phrased it to them that way, that they need protection and need to be aware of what they're doing.

Another issue that has gained a lot of traction in recent years, via the #MeToo movement, is sexual harassment and assault. While parents do need to discuss with their daughters how to stay safe, with my boys, we always had the conversation of a girl's right to say no and treating them respectfully. It's important that both boys and girls are taught appropriate sexual behavior, how to say no, and how to accept no for an answer.

Peer Pressure

Peer pressure is when your child's peers are telling them to do something or to dress a certain way and they don't want to do it. But in order to be accepted in the group, they feel as though they need to.

The bottom line is to give your child coping mechanisms on how to deal with it. That's really the problem. How do you handle that? How do you stand on your own and withstand the pressure? Help them to talk through the problem and develop scripts for how to respond to the pressure.

After Surviving Adolescence …

After adolescence, your children will eventually become full-fledged adults. We'll look at strategies for giving them wings when they are not quite ready to fly and for ensuring the health of your relationship as they take charge of their own lives. ❧

CHAPTER 3

Caring for Adult Children

In your heart, you might always think of your children as your babies. But your relationship with them must grow and change. At some point, they will become full-fledged adults with their own hopes and dreams, thoughts and feelings. And while letting go and encouraging them to be independent is difficult and sometimes counterintuitive, that's exactly what you need to do.

Throughout your child's adult life, your focus must be on maintaining a strong relationship with them, whether they've moved back home or they're on their own and making choices you might not agree with. While you want to be honest with them, you also want to be mindful that how you parented them when they were children no longer applies. The parent-child dynamic must evolve when they become adults.

> ### 💡 FIVE TIPS FOR KEEPING YOUR RELATIONSHIP ON TRACK
>
> - If your child moves home, set ground rules and a timeline.
> - Train yourself not to share petty criticisms.
> - When you do offer advice, be calm, thoughtful, and nonjudgmental.
> - Be up front and clear about what you will and won't help with when it comes to money.
> - Remember that your children are adults with their own identities, not an extension or reflection of you!

"Failure to Launch"

Perhaps your child is struggling with supporting themselves and getting their life started. This is sometimes referred to as "failure to launch." Your adult child might even want to move back home with you! Whether they are living with you or on their own, handling this situation with sensitivity and a clear head will help you and your child to get through it.

WHEN YOUR CHILD MOVES HOME

If your child is in a situation where they just can't take care of themselves—because they've lost a job or because of some other personal problem—you are likely going to want to help out. But there are pitfalls to consider before your child shows up at your house with their belongings.

Most importantly, you have to reestablish rules of the house. It's very unlikely you're going to want to go back to taking care of your child in the same way you did when they were young—doing laundry, cooking meals, cleaning their room, or taking on all of the responsibility for keeping the house running. Returning to this role might be instinctive, but it's not good for either of you, and you're bound to resent the extra burden in the long run.

My advice to parents in this situation is that if you're going to let your child move back in, first set a timeframe for how long the arrangement will last. Acknowledge that you will let them live with you for three months or six months or whatever period you agree is what they need to get back on their feet. Give them a timeline because if they think they can be there forever, they might not be motivated to improve their situation.

Next, establish rules about cooking and cleaning and laundry and so on. Your child should be taking care of their own room and laundry. State your needs when coming up with the rules. Beyond that, decide on household logistics. Who will do the shopping? Who will do the meal preparation? As you assign responsibilities, you might create a schedule for who does what and post it in a common area.

Planning in this manner puts you in the position of not allowing them to return to their childhood habits. These rules make it clear that you're not there to wait on them.

There are exceptions to the rules. I've been involved with cases where the daughter came back home with her children because she was being physically abused by her husband. While you'll still want to define some rules so that you don't return to the parent-as-caregiver role, you probably won't want to set a timeline for the arrangement.

It's also possible that you're both in agreement that you want to live together indefinitely. Your child can live in your house because it might make sense for both of you economically or for some other reason. There's not anything inherently wrong with that. Even so, you will want to come up with a way to live together that distributes the housework and expenses that makes sense for both of you.

TO CHARGE RENT OR NOT TO CHARGE RENT?

If your child returns home, you might want to charge rent, either out of a genuine need to pay for the added costs such as electricity and food or to send the signal that you consider them adults and they need to contribute. Monthly rent might also motivate them to meet their deadlines for moving out.

If you don't need the money, you could set aside what they've contributed for their future needs. My cousin moved home for an extended period, and my uncle charged her rent. He put the money in the bank, and when she got married, he gave it back to her for a deposit for her house.

If you find this idea appealing, you can set up a separate account for this purpose.

> 66
> Think it through ahead of time. Because how you open that discussion is important for setting the tone of the conversation.

WHEN YOUR CHILD'S CAREER FALLS SHORT

Most parents have some sort of a vision for their child's future—some idea of what success will look like for them. Whether that means going to college or settling down and starting a family, we want the best for our children.

Sometimes, though, a child doesn't achieve what you imagined for them. Maybe they are living on their own, but they are just barely able to pay the bills. Or maybe you simply think they are underachieving. Do you say something?

If you're going to have that discussion, think it through ahead of time. Because how you open that discussion is important for setting the tone of the conversation. If you open that discussion with blame or showing disappointment or criticism, it's not going to be productive.

💡 TIP FOR DEALING WITH CONFLICT

There's an old conflict management technique that says to write down what the issues are. If you're both looking at the issues in black and white on paper and not looking at each other eye to eye, sometimes it makes it easier to deal with emotionally charged issues. Looking at neutral territory and not at each other defuses some of the tension.

If you both agree that your child could and should make some sort of career move, you can help them to get some direction. However, I often see parents' expectations that are beyond what their child can achieve. I like to have young adults tested so we all know what they can and can't do. I've seen people be pushed into a four-year college when they really don't belong there. They fail because they need to be in a more appropriate setting for their abilities.

For parents who went to college and are themselves professionals, it can be very hard to move off of the idea of college and to support their child in moving into a trade or some other career that doesn't require a degree. But there are viable, meaningful, skilled careers that don't involve a college education. Maybe it's not what you had in mind, but helping them to get the appropriate training will enable them to support themselves.

I was in a situation recently in which I told the mother that she needed to retrench and ask her son, "What do you really want to do?" She did, and he said, "I would like to be an electrician." This didn't sit well with her, but I told her, "Let him be an electrician."

He made that choice, and he's on the path to a fine career. He's happier, and while she did resist, she's finally getting on board. In the long run, I'm certain that she'll be happier that he's in a profession that suits him and that he's passionate about. It has also improved their relationship. He calls and visits more often as he feels successful and accepted for who he is.

So be realistic about your child's skills and interests and get on board with a plan that makes sense for them. It will pay dividends both in terms of your child's ability to take care of themselves, and by extension, the health of your relationship.

AVOIDING COMPARISONS

Sometimes your child's delays can make you feel embarrassed when you have friends whose children are very successful.

The other parent may or may not be competitive. Maybe they are just proud that their daughter was promoted to VP or just got her medical degree and want to share their happiness with their friends. What do you do?

If you are being bombarded with constant bragging, you may find that this is not someone you want to be with. Just as I did when my son and I were in a playgroup with a super competitive mother, you might need to minimize your time with this person.

What about when you have long-term, good friends who say things like, "My child's doing great," and maybe your child's not doing so great? You might try to make excuses for your child or exaggerate their successes. Resist that urge. Just let it go. Let your friend have their good experience. And you will still love your child and should be proud of the person they have become and their accomplishments. For example, your daughter may be an outstanding and devoted mother or your son a dedicated father and husband or a community volunteer. You get to choose the playing field.

Letting Go

While you might have always imagined your child following in your footsteps—whether it's a career or a lifestyle—you need to learn to support them in their choices. Just as I recommend when your children are young, you need to understand that your children are not a reflection of you. Conversely, while you might be proud of them when they achieve something, realize that it's not your achievement; it's theirs. They are their own people, separate from you, with separate identities! It's hard for a parent to come to terms with this, but it's critical for your relationship—and for their emotional well-being—moving forward.

I often see parents becoming overly invested when their children are athletes. For many years, everything was focused on their being an athlete. If they don't do well in school or they get into a little bit of trouble, as long as they're a starter on the team, life is good. Maybe they'll play in college. But after that, their "career" is done.

I've seen families fall apart over this. They think, "Oh my God, our life is over." But their child has a college degree. They can go on to work and be successful.

It's incredibly unlikely that your child will play professional sports, so you can't live and die on the hope that they'll be picked up by an NFL team or make the US Olympic gymnastics team.

Preventing Estrangement

Many issues can arise that might cause estrangement between you and your adult child. For most parents, their children are the most important people in their lives, so a wedge between you and your child can be devastating. And yet it happens far more often than you'd think. It's important to be sensitive to the types of problems you might face that can cause this type of estrangement.

WHEN YOU DON'T APPROVE OF YOUR CHILD'S PARTNER

Suppose your child becomes engaged to someone you don't like and who you believe won't make a good partner. What do you do?

This is a difficult situation. With the wisdom you've attained through your life experience, maybe you can see problems that make their choice of a partner a poor one. You don't want to stay silent, but saying something might cause a blowout that will result in your child not speaking with you. Estrangements for this reason are not uncommon. How do you walk this tightrope?

One option is to say nothing. This might frustrate you, but unless your child is in physical danger, it might be your only choice if you're to maintain the relationship with your child going forward.

Another option is to have a calm, thoughtful conversation that is not emotionally charged. You can advise your child, pointing out what you are seeing and that you're concerned about it. I would start out with something like, "I am concerned. I am worried, and here's why," as opposed to starting with, "He's a jerk."

I know a mom whose son was seeing a girl she didn't like. A family member asked, "Why don't you do something about it?" And she said, "I've had a conversation with him. I've told him my feelings about this. But in the end, I'm not going to lose my son over a conflict about this relationship."

While it can be frustrating, you need to let go after you've said your piece or risk losing your relationship with your child.

KEEPING MONEY FROM COMING BETWEEN YOU

Money can become an issue in any relationship, whether between you and your spouse, between you and a friend you've loaned money to, or between you and your child. In fact, I know someone who has become estranged from both friends and family members because of her expectations surrounding money.

Know that there is no right and wrong way to provide financial support to your adult children. It is perfectly reasonable to keep your finances separate and expect your child to support themselves without a penny from you. It's also reasonable to loan your child money or to give them a gift for a specific purpose or because you want to start to gift them their inheritance while you are alive if you have a sizeable estate.

Whatever you decide, to keep money from coming between you, be clear about what help you will and will not provide. If you are going to loan your child money, spell out the terms. Also know that it is possible you will never see the money repaid. That's always a risk when you make a personal loan. Are you okay with that? Will it damage your relationship with your child if that happens? These are the matters you need to consider before you become involved financially with your child.

BEING OVERLY CRITICAL

Another thing that causes estrangement is continual criticism of an adult child. Parents sometimes criticize what their child is doing, how they're doing it, how they dress, their weight, what their hair is like, what kind of car they bought, and so on. This sort of constant criticism can do a number on your relationship as well as your child's self-esteem.

Before you speak to your child in this way, think to yourself, "Is this really important? Do I really need to say this?" You have to train yourself to think like that because you're used to saying whatever you want to say to your child. This dynamic might have felt appropriate when they were younger. But now your child's an adult, and your job of intense observation and correction is over.

There's an old Haim Ginott story. Haim Ginott is a psychologist and author of the seminal book *Between Parent and Child*. He tells the story about a friend who comes to visit, and she accidentally leaves her umbrella at your house. You call her up and you say, "Hey, did you realize you left your umbrella at my house?" And she says, "No, I'll come and pick it up."

But if an adult child does the same, what we end up saying is more along the lines of, "You were at the house yesterday, and you left the umbrella again. It's going to rain today. What's wrong with you?"

These are two completely different conversations. What Haim Ginott was saying is that you have to learn to speak to your adult child as you would speak to any other adult. And if you wouldn't say what you're about to say to another adult, then you probably shouldn't be saying it to your child either.

Sometimes it takes a wholesale readjustment of your relationship to make this shift. It's a difficult dynamic to break. But know that it's healthier for you, your child, and your relationship if you can learn to keep your opinions to yourself and let your children live their lives as they see fit.

DIVORCED OR WIDOWED PARENTS AND DATING

Another difficult situation that can come up when your children are adults is your own marriage might fail or your spouse might pass away. After whatever feels like an appropriate waiting period, you might begin to date. This can open up a range of issues with your adult child that could potentially lead to estrangement.

It's possible that your child doesn't want to see you dating at all. When they are unhappy seeing you start to get out there again, you can't appease them by simply not dating. Just as you can't interfere with their adult lives, they don't get a vote in yours!

I have a friend whose twenty-two-year-old son encountered her male visitor when he came to the house. He said to her, "What is this guy doing here? I hope he's not sleeping in your bed." She, very appropriately, said to him, "This is none of your business. This is my life. I'm in my own house, not yours." Fortunately, they made it through that situation. But his initial reaction was very strong.

How you handle this depends on you, your children, and your new relationship. You might choose not to discuss the subject of dating with your children until your relationship gets serious. Then, when it comes time to share details, be sensitive, but know that there is no need to apologize for having your own life and the need for companionship.

On the other hand, sometimes a new relationship can come between a parent and their children. I knew a widowed husband who was dating a woman. Eventually, they became engaged. After the engagement, he wanted to plan a vacation in which he brought his children. His fiancée said no.

There were two possible outcomes from this situation: he could bow to his fiancée's demands, or he could hold his ground. In the end, he decided to end the engagement; his children were more important to him.

Was that the "right" choice? The fact of the matter is there is no single correct answer. I've known people who have separated from their adult children for the sake of a new relationship. Everybody's going to handle this situation differently. But be aware that this is an area where you might need to tread carefully.

> "
> The fact of the matter is there is no single correct answer.

Another aspect of new relationships has to do with money. When you remarry or if you're in a long-term relationship later in life, the issue of money can become very touchy between you and your child. For example, if you remarry, your spouse might be a beneficiary of your estate. Your children might be very unhappy with this and feel they should inherit everything. They also might be very protective of your late spouse's possessions. This can also be an issue if you want to explicitly add some support for your unmarried partner through your will.

The options for how to handle this are endless! I know someone who specified in his will that his spouse could live in their house until she died, and his estate would support her. But after that, his children would inherit the estate. This satisfied both the desire to take care of his new spouse and his children's expectation that they would be his heirs.

In terms of family possessions, if you want your children to have certain items, you can give them to them while you are still alive, or you can stipulate in your will the possessions you want to give to each child.

Ultimately, I can't advise you on how to handle your estate. Your money matters are highly personal and specific to your situation, and I'm not a lawyer. But I *can* advise you to address it by having a will that spells out your wishes; otherwise, your state's inheritance laws will take effect, and this might not be what you want. And while it might be difficult or cause strife between you and your children, I recommend that you let them know ahead of time whether or not they'll inherit that summer home that they always assumed would be theirs.

These are difficult but necessary decisions and conversations.

Your Children's Children

If you're fortunate enough to have grandchildren, you might be put in the role of caregiver for them, either for a short visit or as their guardian. In the next chapter, we'll look at what having grandchildren might mean to you as a caregiver. ❧

CHAPTER 4

Caring for Grandchildren

I'm fortunate not only to have two wonderful grandchildren but to have forged a strong bond with each of them. Given that they don't live nearby, that hasn't happened by accident.

Whether your grandchildren live nearby or far away, you might struggle with developing a relationship with them. Or you might be thrust into the role of caregiver, whether for a few hours or longer term.

The key to building a meaningful relationship with your grandchild is communication—with them and with their parents. And there's a certain art to that, which I've helped many families to put into practice.

> 66
> The key to building a meaningful relationship with your grandchild is communication— with them and with their parents.

Long-Distance Grandparenting

💡 FIVE QUICK TIPS FOR LONG-DISTANCE GRANDPARENTING

With today's technology, you can build and maintain a relationship with your grandchildren over a distance and between visits. So ...

1. Take full advantage of the technology. Having a Zoom call? Simply talking to a young child over Zoom or FaceTime can be boring and sometimes even confusing for them. Be prepared with something specific to share with them: a song, puppets, or a story to read.

2. Play games together, even with older children. What are their interests? Follow their lead. There are many online games and apps that allow for multiple players. An ongoing connection via games like Words with Friends, for example, can help to strengthen your bond.

3. Form a "book club" in which you read the same book and then meet to talk about it. Different opinions are a positive in this setting, making for an engaging conversation.

4. Get moving! Try exercising or dancing together. Yoga and other fitness classes are plentiful online. Or you can make up your own dances and even make a TikTok video together.

5. Encourage your grandchildren to share their schoolwork with you, to show you their test papers, their artwork ... whatever is important to them.

On the AARP website, the subject that comes up the most is long-distance grandparenting. Regardless of economic status, seniors want to know how to have relationships with grandchildren when they don't see them. Sometimes, even if they live two hours away, they might not see them very often. Having a strong relationship when you are long distance takes some effort.

I was in this situation when my grandchildren were living in New York, and I was in Ohio. I was able to fly to New York once a month so I could be with them, but not everyone can manage trips like that. However, you can see your grandchildren infrequently and still build strong relationships with them.

When my grandchildren were very young, I found that the best way to form and maintain a long-distance relationship with them was through songs that we sang together. I sang them special songs that my grandmother and mother sang to me and new songs, such as "Take Me Out of the Bathtub," which I learned from a book of children's songs. Singing these songs together provided us with an immediate connection even when I couldn't travel and visit with them for a month or two. (I find that the more dramatic you are when singing the more memorable the experience is—and lots of fun!)

Another way you can do that is to write good, old-fashioned letters. That's what I did, especially when my grandchildren were first learning to read. I made it fun by occasionally using stickers in place of words. For example, if I wrote, "I heard you were at the beach," I would place a sticker of something that had to do with the beach. They loved to receive letters from their grandma.

Another way to build a relationship is to follow their lead when you're with them rather than trying to press your interests on them. See the movies they want to see, read what they're reading, watch their TV show with them. That'll give you something to talk about that they are interested in.

While these techniques can help, research shows that the best and deepest relationships with children are formed around play. Playing can take many forms. If you don't necessarily like to play games but you love to cook, when you do see them, they can be in the kitchen working side by side with you, stirring or measuring out ingredients, for example.

Your grandchildren can also come to visit you, with or without their parents. I took my grandchildren whenever the opportunity arose. The one-on-one time with them was invaluable. Sometimes I would visit there and encourage my son and daughter-in-law to go for a night or two on the town—my treat. It was good for them, good for the grandchildren and me, and as a bonus, good for my relationship with my son and his wife.

Gifts

One of the joys of grandparenting can be giving your grandchildren gifts. The types of gifts that you give will depend on the age of the child. When a child is young, I recommend that you not give toys that make a lot of loud and constant noise. Remember that, when you leave, that noisy, annoying toy is still going to be there. It's fun for the children but annoying for the parents. Drums, loud sirens, and blaring noise are not great gifts as far as the parents are concerned. Don't give anything that will be annoying in the household. Such toys can become a point of conflict when the child wants to play with it and the parent doesn't want to hear that noise anymore.

Often, grandparents don't know what gifts to give, especially with older children. You can always give cash, but that's not as meaningful as something they can hold in their hand (although it might be exactly what they want!). A cash gift doesn't build a memory that they'll carry forward. If you are stuck as to what to get, ask their parents what they want or at least get some ideas as to what they're into at the moment. You can also ask other grandparents what they've given to their grandchildren that has gone over well. If you give them something they've wanted or that's up their alley, they will remember it—and you—for the rest of their lives.

Conversely, if you know your grandchildren's parents are opposed to their having certain things, don't be the one to supply it against their wishes. Whether or not you agree with them, if they don't want them to have the latest Xbox, for example, don't buy it. If you know your adult children are opposed to something and they don't want your grandchildren to have it, then this is not the time to step over a line. That object is going to stay in their house, and they're going to deal with it. Or they're going to take it away, and you've bought an expensive gift that's not going to get used.

Instead, have a discussion with the parents and say, "Here are some gift ideas I'm thinking about. What do you think?"

When you do give a gift, I would advise that you not tell your grandchild how much it cost. I know someone whose grandchildren came back from a day of shopping with their grandmother. The grandson told his parents that his grandmother spent a large amount of money on him that day. They asked, "How do you know that?" And he said, "Because she told me. She always tells me how much she's spending on me."

That sort of interaction doesn't make for a great relationship.

Gifts that have sentimental value can be more important and meaningful than expensive gifts. For example, for my granddaughter's Bat Mitzvah, I didn't want to give her cash. Then I realized that I have a really beautiful necklace that she would like. It was the last gift that my husband gave me before he passed away. And there was a story behind this gift about how he had to get his caregiver to take him to the jewelry shop without my knowing.

I realized that these kinds of opportunities are a time to start giving things away that have meaning. I wrote a letter about my husband and how he bought the necklace, what it meant to him, and how he loved his family. When I gave her this necklace, we read the letter together, and we had a touching moment. Then she wore the necklace for her Bat Mitzvah.

She wrote me the loveliest thank-you note and explained that she felt that, in a way, we had Grandpa with us at the Bat Mitzvah. This gift had a lot more meaning than if I'd bought her something.

Special occasions are an opportunity to begin to give some things away to your grandchildren. And when you can still talk about the story or meaning behind it and share that with them, it's extra special.

Discipline

You might be in a position in which you feel you need to apply some discipline to your grandchildren. The main thing I recommend with grandparents in this case is *not to undermine your adult children*. (The exception is if their disciplinary techniques are abusive, in which case, you'll need to intercede.)

If you disagree with what they are doing, you can always have a conversation privately, away from the children. Otherwise, do not interfere; that will backfire on you. If you want to discipline the grandchildren in a different way, you can do it when the grandchildren are alone with you.

The parents might worry that using different styles of disciple might confuse the children. But children adapt easily. They understand that there's a different set of rules depending on who they're with. I once had a situation when my grandson was very young, and he wanted something that I told him that he couldn't have. He started crying and screaming. My granddaughter, who's three years older, said to him, "Just stop it. You're dealing with the wrong grandparent." The tears dried up instantly because he knew that this grandma didn't respond to that.

Very often, grandparents are given specific instructions about what to do or what not to do in terms of discipline. My tack with that (assuming the child's safety was not at stake), if I didn't agree with it or it was clearly not important, was to say, "Uh-huh." And then, when the parents weren't there, I did what felt natural to me that worked.

However, when a practice was a part of that child's routine, I felt I did really need to follow it because getting them out of the routine was going to cause a problem.

Suppose you're doing something that the parents are really opposed to, and they tell you, "Please, don't do that." At that point, you really have to listen. Especially if they don't want the child to have sweets—either because of their weight or because of how active they get when they return home—you really must follow their instructions.

Sometimes they might say something like, "We're having problems with John right now because he's not getting enough sleep. We've laid down the rule that he has to turn off all electronics an hour before bedtime." That's an established routine, so you have to abide by that.

On the other hand, the parents need to understand that one night with Grandma being a little too permissive is not going to be the end of the world if there were other benefits (like a night off for them!).

Bridging the Generation Gap

There might be fifty, sixty, or even seventy years or more between you and your grandchildren. While you might keep up with the latest trends and technology, there are bound to be generational differences in the way you think and communicate.

For example, my grandchildren are in the generation where pronouns have become important. This is a concept my generation is not familiar with, and I have found that I need to be very careful about how I respond. When my granddaughter told me her teacher wants to be referred to with they/them pronouns, I was genuinely puzzled. Your reaction to changes that are going on in their world and the world around them can cause issues with your grandchild.

As your grandchildren get older, they start to have very strong opinions about trends, technology, and politics. I overheard a grandparent say, "My grandchild feels really strongly about a political issue. And I told her, 'That's a bunch of crap.'" And I was thinking, "I understand you may disagree. But there's a better way of communicating that you disagree." You have to be very careful because you can close down communication.

If you feel you can't have a conversation on the topic without it becoming too fiery, you can affirm their feelings without agreeing with them. You can say something along the lines of, "You must feel passionately about that" or "That's great that you're becoming politically involved."

Sometimes, I give my grandchildren my opinion and explain why I feel that way. For instance, when Lily told me about her teacher, I said, "I am having difficulty with that because to me they/them is a plural, and she's a singular person. It's a disconnect for me based on what I learned about grammar growing up."

She understood that. But young people have a very negative reaction If you say something along the lines of, "That's crap, and I disagree with it." Instead, I find that when you give them a reason, and you explain why you're having difficulty with understanding it, they may not agree with you, but they can at least enter into a calm discussion.

Communication

As I mentioned earlier, communication is key to maintaining healthy relationships with your grandchildren. This communication includes the people around your grandchildren, such as their parents and even the other set of grandparents.

Before your grandchild is even born, it's a good idea to sit down and talk to the expectant parents about what your version of grandparenting will look like. The following script encapsulates how I think grandparenting should go.

> "There are many ways to raise a successful child, so I'm not going to interfere. If I come to you to talk to you about something about my grandchildren, it's going to be because I consider it to be extremely important. Otherwise, I'm not going to say anything to you. If your daughter walks outside, and I think it's cold and she needs to put a jacket on, I'm not saying anything. If I disagree with what you're feeding her, I'm not saying anything. That's between you and your child's pediatrician. If I *do* come to you, it's going to be because I consider it to be a very serious, critical issue."

And then you have to be willing to live with that and abide by it.

KEEPING IT POSITIVE

A GOOD WORD FROM THE GRANDPARENTS

In my practice as a therapist, I have worked with many families in which grandparents were deeply involved. As a result of this work,

I developed a therapeutic technique called *Intergenerational Play Therapy*. One aspect of this technique was for the grandparents to tell the therapist what went well in the last week. That becomes their job: watch for what is going well. Find the positives and comment on them.

Grandparents can either support or undermine change in the family. For example, in therapy I might recommend that the parents change the way a child is disciplined. Sometimes the grandparents undermine changes because they take these changes as a personal affront to their own parenting techniques. They get very angry, and they start to undermine the changes in the family.

So, I change their role to one of noticing what went well. And in forcing them to really observe what went well and what was positive, it changes the whole relationship and the family dynamics. But they have to understand that that is their role: to observe, point out, and talk about what's going well.

In the technique I developed, when there is friction in the family and they come to me for help, I retrain the grandparents to focus on spotting the positive. When they came into therapy, my first question to them is "What went well this week?" I developed this technique because the tendency is to note all the negatives. It's human nature.

If eventually you want to get to speaking about the negative, you have to start with a positive, like, "Wow, this was a great meal" or "The kids look terrific" or "You're working so hard. I don't know how you do it."

What comes out of your mouth for a period of time has to be positive. People get used to you being positive and they appreciate it. Then, if a concern comes up, they will listen. That's what happened with me when I noticed something I thought might be concerning about my grandson. It was unusual for me to say, "I'm concerned about something" or make a comment other than a positive one, so when I did have something to say, the parents were receptive.

I've seen grandparents who were constantly criticizing and harping on things and seeing things that weren't there. I knew someone whose mother-in-law was highly critical, and she couldn't take it anymore. She told her mother-in-law, "I can't take this anymore. If we're leaving the house, and the baby doesn't have a hat on, you've got to calm down and stop making such a big deal out of it." The mother-in-law said, "Fine." What she did instead was she started to talk to the mom as if she were speaking for the baby. If they were leaving the house, she would say something like, "Oh Mommy! I think it's so cold out. Maybe I need a hat." This was just as bad, if not worse!

As a grandparent, try to limit your comments on the raising of your grandchildren. You did what you wanted to do when you were parenting. Likely, your parents did not always agree with everything you were doing, either, and you probably didn't care for their interference. You, too, need to keep your criticism to yourself as much as possible. Sit back and think through your own experiences as a parent and the kinds of things that were said to you by your own parents or other family members that were not helpful.

Remember, too, that, as a grandparent, it's not your goal to raise the children. Personally, I feel that I've raised my children already. My goal now is to enjoy my grandchildren, and, if I see something that worries me, be able to communicate that. I'm not going to accomplish that by constantly nitpicking and criticizing things that aren't important.

If I *am* going to say something, I start out with, "I am concerned" or "I'm a little worried and wanted to share this with you." Don't say things like, "I've looked at John, and he's really a mess." That isn't helpful.

COMMUNICATING WITH YOUR CHILD ABOUT THE GRANDCHILDREN

Communicating with your children about their parenting takes just a little bit of common sense.

First and foremost, respect their decisions even if you disagree. This is especially true with daughters, who appear to be much more sensitive to opinions about their parenting styles and skills. It's important to be aware of their feelings about being a good mother. Prior to making a comment, take a breath and think:

- Is what I'm going to say really necessary?

- What will be the impact?

While the role of men in parenting is constantly changing and evolving, there is still an assumption in many cases that the mom is the primary caregiver. So, it can only help when you reinforce her positive behaviors, such as playing with the children, helping out around the house, and giving back to the community. Make sure to tell her what a wonderful mother you think she is and how much she means to you.

COMMUNICATING WITH YOUR IN-LAW CHILDREN

Speaking to your in-law child is different from speaking with your own child. However, the same principles apply as with your own child. Support their decisions unless you believe the consequences will be detrimental to the family.

Daughters-in-law tend to be a little more sensitive. I find young women these days often feel a sense of disloyalty to their own mothers through forming a close relationship with their mother-in-law. In these circumstances, forming a relationship with your daughter-in-law takes time and patience. Don't pressure her or push the relationship too fast. Give it time.

Also, make the effort to give compliments to your daughter-in-law about her parenting. Most importantly, be tactful.

> ### 💡 TIP FOR GETTING AN IMPORTANT MESSAGE THROUGH TO YOUR GRANDCHILDREN'S PARENTS
>
> Sometimes your in-law child will be more receptive to what you're saying about your grandchildren than your own child, if you have a good relationship with them. It might be easier to broach the matter with them. Sometimes they are the better pathway for communication about a serious matter that you believe needs to be attended to.

COMMUNICATING WITH THE OTHER GRANDPARENTS

Sometimes there's a conflict between you and the other mother-in-law or father-in-law. This is particularly problematic if you have to see them frequently. If you can see them three or four times a year, it's best to learn to keep quiet as best you can and live with the occasional stress of seeing them.

If you do see them more often, one approach is to limit your conversation with them. If you need to communicate outside of in-person social gatherings, try texting instead of talking.

Know that your interactions with the other set of grandparents are being watched by your daughter-in-law or son-in-law and your grandchildren. How you interact with them influences these relationships. Try to keep things positive and friendly even if you are gritting your teeth because you really don't like them and the things they say. It's hard on the grandchildren or the children when something negative is being said about someone they love. And it doesn't end up hurting the person they love when you do that; it hurts you, and it hurts your relationship. When you voice your negative thoughts, you're seen as the bad guy.

💡 HOT TIP: BE COOL ABOUT YOUR IN-LAW'S PARENTS

How you treat your daughter-in-law's or son-in-law's parents can make a difference in your relationship with your daughter-in-law or son-in-law, as well as your son or daughter.

Suppose your daughter-in-law is fighting with her mother. That's fine. That's normal. Tempting as it may be, don't join in! If you start being negative or fighting with her mother, that's not going to be good for your relationships with your daughter-in-law and your son.

Grandparenting during a Divorce

Divorce becomes complicated when grandparents take sides and especially when a lot of money is involved. When this happens, everyone loses their focus on what's happening with the children.

It's natural to take the side of your child and look out for your child's financial welfare. However, your most important role is to remind the parents to think about what is in the best interest of the children and keep them focused on that. Don't get involved in what's going on otherwise unless you have some sort of expertise that your child relies on. And when possible, try to be supportive to your child's partner.

I've treated kids in therapy, so I've heard a lot of what was very disruptive to them. So, for example, if your child is trying to get a custody or visitation arrangement out of anger or spite that is clearly not in the best interest of the children, your role is to steer them toward what's best for the children rather than helping to feed that anger.

You might be concerned that you'll become estranged from your grandchildren, especially if your child does not have primary custody and you don't have the best relationship with your son-in-law or daughter-in-law. Even if everything is okay between you now, you can't guess what the future will bring, say if one of the partners remarries or has a committed relationship.

That happens a lot, which is why I usually recommend that families use a mediator when trying to settle a divorce. As part of their separation agreement, the parents should work out a vacation schedule—who's going to have the children and when—and put it in writing. In the course of these negotiations, they'll determine who has the kids for each holiday and who sees them for various long weekends and vacations.

Once the schedule is worked out, you'll see where you figure into that. If the grandchildren live close by, it will probably be easier to get time with them on the weekends your child has them.

Whether you live in the same area or you're doing a weekly Zoom call, you might have an uncooperative child-in-law who wants to restrict your access. My theory is to hang out a lot and be quiet. Because when you do that, people talk to you. (I gave this same advice with regard to adolescents.) Suppose one of the spouses is having an affair, and the other spouse is really angry and vindictive. You need to keep quiet and try to be very supportive of that other person, and again, stay focused on the children. When you do have an opportunity to express yourself, here's a sample script:

> "I understand this is really hard for you, and you're really angry, but it's not going to help the situation for you to cut off my contact or communication with the children. They have a close relationship with me, and the divorce will be even harder on them if that relationship is terminated."

It's all in the approach, and the quiet, more passive approach works better. Starting conversations with, "Look, we need to discuss this" with an in-law just doesn't work. I suggest starting out conversations with, "I love you. I love the grandchildren. You're a wonderful mom. I'm very sad about thinking that I would lose my connection to the children." That opening is a lot different and more productive.

On the other hand, I know of two situations where the grandparents have sued to have access to the grandchildren. That's the extreme, but it happens. This might happen when the situation is absolutely unworkable, no matter what you say or do. If you're dealing with someone who's unreasonable, then it's very rare you can get them back on track.

What if you didn't have much of a relationship with the grandchildren before the divorce? The divorce is not a time to change things. If you have not been very involved with the kids, this is not the time to suddenly offer to take them. Whatever the status quo is at that point, maintain it.

One more thing: It's very important to maintain an amicable relationship with your in-law's parents (the other grandparents) if at all possible. People forget that you're all going to end up in the same place at the same time for an event like a wedding or a graduation or a birthday party. If you've closed that door by saying negative or angry things that you can never take back, those family events will always be a time of conflict.

WHAT TO DO WITH YOUR STRONG EMOTIONS ABOUT THE DIVORCE

I've been recommending that you keep your thoughts to yourself throughout your child's divorce. But you're going to have strong feelings. You can have your feelings, but you have to be careful who you express them to.

Most people have at least one trusted friend or a family member who will not repeat what they're saying. While you'll want to be careful not to reveal all the personal things that are going on with your child, it's okay to vent and get it out. Better to a friend and not to your child, your in-law child, or your grandchildren.

Grandparenting Is Different from Parenting!

It's possible that your child might not want you to spend much time with your grandchildren. Maybe you didn't have the best parent-child relationship, and your child doesn't trust you to be with their children. (If there's a history of abuse, that's understandable, and that distance should be maintained.)

But I find that some people who were not necessarily the best parents often make great grandparents. Perhaps as parents you were working long hours or were experiencing pressure from your own parents. As a grandparent, your life is often different and less stressful. Take Frank, my husband. He was a great father, but he was very strict. The kids would ask for things, and he would put them through a financial grilling. "Do we really *need* this? Or do we *want* it? And what if we saved up your allowance so you had to pay for it?" He was taking his role of parenting seriously and trying to teach the children important life skills.

But I'll never forget the first time we took our granddaughter to a Broadway show to see *Mary Poppins*. She was very young, and she pointed to the Mary Poppins paraphernalia, and said, "Ooh, I'd like to have that Mary Poppins doll." My husband said, "Of course. Just point to anything you want for Grandpa, and I'll get it for you. Whatever you want."

Grandparents as Primary Caregivers

A GREAT RESOURCE FOR GRANDPARENTS

If you are raising your grandchildren, you can find a comprehensive list of resources at https://ncrc.org/resources-for-grandparents-raising-grandchildren/.

Sometimes, when a parent has a serious problem—typically drug addiction—a child is placed with their grandparents. Caring for your grandchildren by acting as their parents can be an exhausting experience for which you need respite and support.

There are many good resources out there for grandparents in this situation (see *Resources for Grandparents*). Beyond those, grandparents often form their own support groups. Check with your local houses of worship or community or senior center to see if there is one in your area.

What happens when your child has recovered and is capable of raising the children? If the transition is to happen, it's in the grandchildren's best interest to make that transition go as smoothly as possible.

In these situations, the biggest issue is trust. You are probably very protective of the grandchildren and have a lack of trust in your child to parent. I often see grandparents making that transition very difficult, which creates a lot of conflict. Both you and your child need to move slowly and in stages to rebuild that trust.

I also see grandparents who have gained legal guardianship use that guardianship as a threat or a weapon. Suppose the parent takes the child back and starts to date someone the grandparent doesn't like. The grandparent might say something like, "Remember, I still have legal guardianship. If you continue your relationship with that person, I'll go back into court and take your child away from you."

We tell the grandparent that the goal is to reunite their adult child with their grandchild and to support their adult child in becoming a responsible parent. It's not helpful to threaten whenever something doesn't go your way or you see something you don't like. Unless the child's well-being is at stake, threatening to use legal guardianship as leverage to take that child away is a maneuver I do not recommend. Chances are, you will lose both the grandchild and your adult child, and then you will have no way to monitor what's going on.

Caring for Specific Family Members

In the next several chapters, I'll talk about the specific issues you might be dealing with when taking care of your spouse or partner, a parent or other senior, or your child. ❧

CHAPTER 5

Caring for a Spouse or Partner

When something unexpected happens to your spouse's or partner's health, it can turn your life upside down. I know this not only because of what I'm exposed to in my work but because it happened to me when my husband, Frank, suddenly became very ill. We went from living a normal life to requiring around-the-clock care for him in our home.

I understand both from a professional standpoint and firsthand what's helpful when caring for a partner. I also know what's *not* helpful and how to overcome some of the adversity you might be facing.

Your Feelings

Before we dig into the practicalities of caring for a spouse or partner, let's talk about how you might be feeling. You might feel a range of emotions, from anger to remorse, from guilt and fear to resentment.

Very often, I hear caregivers resist facing their feelings about their situation. And they certainly don't tell anyone because we believe that, as caregivers, we are expected to be caring people. We may be tired but never resentful or angry. But denying those feelings can make caregiving even more difficult.

DEALING WITH RESENTMENT

Sometimes there's a history in which an ill spouse was not kind to you, and now you're their caregiver. It's hard to provide care when you feel that you have been mistreated. In fact, I knew a woman whose husband told her he was going to leave her, but then he had a stroke before he moved out. The wife felt obliged to provide care for him at home until her children were grown. That was a very tough situation for her.

> I would also encourage you to find time to engage in your stress relievers, whatever they may be.

Maybe your partner wasn't nice to you or didn't make any effort to take care of you when they were healthy. If you were sick, maybe they wouldn't even bring you a cup of tea. You might be filled with resentment that now you have to devote yourself to caring for them when, if the roles were reversed, they wouldn't do the same for you.

These are real emotions, and they're okay to have.

What do you with your anger or resentment?

You have a few options, and any combination of these outlets can help. One is to see a professional so you can divulge everything you are feeling in confidence and without fear of judgment. Another is to vent to a trusted friend.

I would also encourage you to find time to engage in your stress relievers, whatever they may be. For example, get on the treadmill, take a walk, or take yourself out for dinner.

How do you get yourself out? If you're using a home health aide or an adult day health center, take advantage of that time to remove yourself from the situation for a bit. See if you can find a friend to come visit your partner for a bit while you take a walk around the neighborhood. Getting out at least a couple of times a week can decrease your intense emotions significantly.

MOURNING, GRIEVING, AND REGRETS

When your loved one is incapacitated by illness, there's usually a mourning and grieving process. I can't tell you how many families I speak to who say, "We had really planned out our retirement" or "We were going to take trips and volunteer together," and now that's not going to happen. Whatever the couple envisioned, together or as individuals, has been lost. So, even though your partner may still be with you, you'll likely find yourself going through a mourning process. That is a necessary step.

I also see people drive themselves crazy wondering whether they could have prevented the illness or health crisis. They wonder if they should have taken their spouse to the doctor sooner or made them stick to their diet better. But in the end, you need to realize that everyone is responsible for themselves.

My own husband had weight issues that were impacting his

health. I was concerned and convinced him to enter a program in which he lost a lot of weight. But, when he became ill, he began eating unhealthily and gained weight again, which impacted his recovery.

I look back on it and say, maybe I should have been more forceful. Maybe I should have made him stay on his diet. But in the end, he was going to have his way. If he wanted a chocolate bar, he would get his caregivers to bring it to him. That's just how it was.

I came to realize that some things are not within my control. Maybe others will try to hold you responsible for your spouse's actions, but the fact remains that he or she is an adult, and you can't make them comply with your wishes. Your spouse is not your child.

FORGIVENESS: FOR THEM AND FOR YOURSELF

When people are ill, they feel their own emotions. They sometimes tend to be a little short tempered, impatient, and demanding. When that happens, you have to try to find it within yourself to understand that and forgive them in order to go forward.

Dementia poses a particular set of challenges. When you're healthy, on a regular basis you might think a negative thought— something even a little mean!—but you don't say it because you know it's hurtful. That's what I call a *filter*. With dementia, though, people lose their filter. You end up seeing their bare emotions.

Without a filter, your loved one might go ahead and say whatever they're thinking. The wife of a client with dementia told me, "My husband was sitting at the kitchen table and said, 'Hey, dummy, why don't you get dinner on already?' He's never spoken to me like that." Chances are, he's thought something along those lines before. We all think mean or even cruel thoughts; without the filter, these thoughts are exposed. It's part of the illness, so try not to hold it against them.

Not only is forgiving your partner important, but it's also important that you forgive yourself for being a less-than-perfect caregiver. For example, with Frank, if I had only two or three hours of sleep, I wasn't always the most patient person in the morning. After Frank passed away, I thought, "I should have been nicer in the morning. I should have smiled and said, 'Good morning, sunshine,' but I was exhausted." I wasn't mean, but I wasn't as kind to him as I could have been.

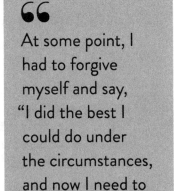

> 66
> At some point, I had to forgive myself and say, "I did the best I could do under the circumstances, and now I need to move on."

At some point, I had to forgive myself and say, "I did the best I could do under the circumstances, and now I need to move on."

Family Events

An issue you might face with friends or family members happens when there's been what we call a change of status. For example, maybe a stroke was involved, or cognitively they're getting worse. I find that if you're going to, say, Thanksgiving dinner, or you're going to a wedding or some other family event, it's best to talk with the family beforehand and paint the picture of what this person's capabilities are, rather than just showing up with them. If you are going to a larger family event, consider bringing someone to help you. Bringing a home care or adult day health center aide might allow you and your partner to be more relaxed and enjoy having time together.

Who's Caring for You?

Caregiving can be exhausting, and you're bound to need a break—a respite from your seemingly never-ending duties. A respite might mean running a particular errand, but it also might mean just having a nap or taking a walk to reenergize yourself.

TAKE A NAP!

Caregivers sometimes think that if they're finally going to take respite that it has to be for a reason, like going to a doctor's appointment or to the bank or taking care of something specific. But maybe you just need to go home and take a nap or read a book. Sleep is so important when you're in a situation in which you are the one providing care. Please know that it's not just okay to allow yourself some relaxation and rest; it's necessary.

GETTING SOME RESPITE

Here are a few ways you might get some respite.

- Regularly bring your loved one to an adult day health center.

- Hire a home health aide.

- Take friends and family up on offers to help.

While it can be difficult to accept help from friends and family, you may find sincere offers coming your way. *Before* that happens, I recommend that you have at the ready a list of things that you need help with. That way, if someone asks, you have an answer.

A MESSAGE TO FAMILY AND FRIENDS

Friends and family members might feel obliged to offer to help you, and that's great if they have the fortitude to do so. On the other one hand, I say to these well-intentioned people: if you really don't want to help, you're uncomfortable helping, or you can't help, then don't make the offer. You might be uncomfortable coming into the house if the patient has Alzheimer's disease, especially if you are close with them. Or if they have cancer and your mother had cancer, for example, you might feel traumatized as you relive your parent's difficult illness.

It's okay if you can't deal with it. But if that's the case, don't make an offer that you are not able to fulfill.

Adult Day Health Centers

Adult day health centers operate during the daytime and provide a range of care and activities. Some centers are open seven days a week, while others are open five or six days. The hours of operation vary as well. Some might be open just a few hours a day, while some, like ours, are open most of the day.

There are two reasons for sending your partner to an adult day health center: the therapies they offer and the respite they give you.

THERAPEUTIC VISITS

An adult day health center can offer activities that can be helpful to ill adults, such as dementia patients. Depending on the offerings of the center, the patient can get stimulation, and for dementia patients, reality orientation.

An adult day health center can also help to get the person out of the isolation. In the medical models like ours, the nurses monitor their health on a regular basis. They become part of their healthcare team. They're making sure the patient is eating and they're reviewing their meds. And they might also be able to provide personal care, such as showers.

How often should you bring your spouse or partner to an adult day health center? The research shows that they have to attend a minimum of two days a week. Otherwise, they don't get into a routine, they don't form relationships, and the staff doesn't get to know them as well.

While a home health aide can be helpful, depending on the quality of the provider, I find that adult day health centers provide better healthcare, and it's better for the patients psychologically and cognitively. When you're home all the time, you tend to get sloppy in the way you dress. You don't put on your makeup anymore. You don't comb your hair. You don't realize what day it is, and you start getting more tired because you're not going out.

Even for someone with dementia, when we force them to go out, they become more oriented. Mentally, it touches something within them that they want to get dressed, and they are suddenly concerned about their appearance.

The other nice thing about these centers is that the staff is available to the family to give them care suggestions that work. Very often we say, especially to a husband, "Take all the clothes out of the closet. If you want her to have a choice, you need to just put in four articles of clothing, so she doesn't get overwhelmed. Take out all that makeup. Just leave two or three things, and then she can remain a little more independent."

Those kinds of suggestions can be very helpful when they come from knowledgeable professionals.

RESPITE FOR THE CAREGIVER

The primary reason why people go into a nursing home early is because of the health of the family caregiver. Sleep deprivation and stress can take years off of you, and you could be in danger of no longer being able to care for your spouse. That's another reason why respite for the caregiver is so important.

I'm familiar with every option in the continuum of adult care. I prefer adult day health centers for respite because it gets the patient out. It cuts through the isolation and depression. At the same time, the nurses are there to monitor their healthcare, so they can intervene before an issue becomes a problem.

I find this option better than most home care in which someone comes in because, usually, they don't provide any structure or an escape from isolation.

WHO CAN GO AND HOW IS IT PAID FOR?

Adult day health centers can be covered by Medicaid and by the Veterans Administration (VA). Some of the long-term health insurance policies will also cover it.

While there's no age restriction to adult day health centers, there are funding restrictions. Sometimes the funding doesn't begin until age sixty or sixty-two. If you're dealing with Medicaid, in some states there are age restrictions. For the VA, the restrictions have to do with service connectedness and the assessment in the VA center about the services they need.

Some centers specialize in younger people. These patients usually have a traumatic brain injury, either from the military or from vehicular accidents. Some have multiple sclerosis (MS) or have needed care throughout their lives. But there are some centers that will take in younger people along with older people.

A younger adult—someone in their forties, say—has other funding source options. Title IV funding applies to those under sixty. For this population, if the funding is in place, my concern becomes whether they fit into the center. We've had some forty-year-olds with MS, for example, who do well in the centers. They adapt, and they love it. And we've had some forty-year-olds who do not adapt. In that case, we've had to help families find some other type of care for them.

When to Involve Your Adult Children

When your spouse is ill, when do you include your adult children in the decision-making process?

To a large extent, it depends on your relationship with your children and where they live. If none of them live close to you, most likely you will be informing them and keeping them in the loop rather than trying to get their buy-in on treatment plans.

If the children haven't seen the person you're caring for, they won't have a good concept of what's happening. This might create conflict in the family. In that case, you might want to have a family meeting, but I recommend doing so face to face so they can see what's really going on.

In a crisis, you might not have time to include the children in the decisions. When I had to make a life-or-death decision about my husband, one son was there, and I got my other son on the phone. We all spoke to the doctor at the same time. Using that approach, everybody gets to ask their questions and hear the physician's answer at the same time.

Friends and Family

As far as your spouse's siblings or other family members go, while you can share information with them and listen to input, I don't recommend giving everyone a vote. At some point, you have to make decisions based on your relationship with your spouse. You can invite their family members to, say, be on the call with the physician or be in the meeting if they live in the area. You can extend that invitation. But in the end, it has to be your decision, and you have to feel confident and set boundaries with them.

On the other hand, I find that, in the end, most people don't want to make important health decisions for their siblings. They're usually happier to have you take control and make the decisions.

UNSOLICITED OPINIONS

Everyone has an opinion about what you should be doing, how you should be doing it, who you should be talking to, and which doctor you should be using. In the end, you have to trust yourself, and you have to trust your own opinion. And you can't interpret other people's opinions as being criticisms of you. People suggest something to someone, sometimes trying to be helpful, but the other person interprets it as a criticism. And then they just block it, and they don't listen.

Sometimes people are trying to be helpful and actually, if you listen to them, sometimes they have useful information, especially if they've been through it or they know really good professionals, facilities, or caregivers to recommend. But if you block them because you interpret everything as a criticism, then you'll never hear it.

Concerned friends and family members need to be careful how they word their suggestions. There are a lot of sentence starters that are very triggering, like the following.

"Why don't you ... "
"If I were you ... "
"Look, don't be upset, but ... "

These phrases can make you angry, so it's hard to listen to the rest of that sentence.

It's more helpful when someone asks, "Are you aware of this resource?" or if they say, "I know someone who was in a similar situation. I can put you in touch with them if that's helpful." If it's possible to calmly lead the conversation to avoid the triggering expressions, try a script like the following.

I understand you are trying to be helpful, but when you push an opinion on me without being in my shoes, it's hard for me to hear. If you have some resources to offer, I'd like to hear about them if you can provide them in a less confrontational way.

Finances

I can't tell you how many families have lost lots of money because their spouse or partner who they shared finances with either has dementia or is ill and receiving treatment. They might have gotten confused and stopped handling things well.

When your spouse or partner has an immediate diagnosis that may affect them cognitively, one of the first steps I recommend is to speak to your lawyer. You may need to get accounts moved— quickly—if they are not already in your name.

You also might have to be concerned about paying the bills. When you're sharing finances, your partner's incapacitation might result in your taking over the bills for the first time. Maybe that's something that you can do, or maybe that's something that you need help with. Sometimes elder services have volunteers who can help with that, or maybe you have a child who can be helpful in this situation.

You might need to obtain power of attorney so you can pay bills and have access to accounts that are not joint ones.

In my situation, Frank had certain accounts that I was not on top of. We segregated those funds, and I lost track of them. Once he got really ill, I had to go through our tax returns and figure it all out and stop automatic investments from happening. It was quite difficult, and I needed help to untangle. Looking back, I probably should have remained engaged in case anything happened.

Another Adult to Care For

While there are very different emotions involved in caring for a parent than for a partner, the logistics may be similar if you are caring for your parent in your home. In the next chapter, we'll look at the issues that arise that are specific to caring for one or both of your parents, in or out of your home. 🕊

CHAPTER 6

Caring for Parents

Taking care of a parent can involve a range of emotions and skills, depending on your parent's health, where they are living, your relationship with them and your siblings, and other factors. They might be in their own home, in an assisted living facility, or you might be caring for them in your home. Regardless of the situation, caring for an aging or ill parent can be challenging.

While caring for a parent can differ from caring for your partner or spouse, many of the issues that arise when you care for a spouse—particularly a spouse with dementia—also arise when caring for an aging parent. So, I recommend that you also read "Chapter 5: Caring for a Spouse or Partner" in addition to "Chapter 8: Common Issues for Providing Healthcare" if you haven't already.

Emotions

Feelings for parents can be complex, and you are apt to have some strong emotions if you find yourself in the role of their caregiver.

ANGER OR RESENTMENT

When caring for a parent, you might have lingering feelings of anger or resentment toward them. I deal with people all the time who say things like, "My father was abusive to me, and suddenly I have to take care of him," or "My mother was really mean and neglectful, and now I'm expected to take her into my home." How do you handle these feelings?

When you feel this way, but you are in a position where you really need to be involved in the care, it might be a good time to make amends and try to resolve the issues. You might have to come to terms with what they did, and in some cases, acknowledge that they did the best they could do at the time. Either you need to be able to talk about it, make amends, and forgive them, or you need to turn over their care to someone else. Because staying in conflict daily doesn't work for you, and it doesn't work for them.

I've dealt with people whose parents were abusive—sometimes physically abusive, sometimes emotionally abusive. And I say the same thing to all of them: "You're at a decision point. Either turn over the care to someone else or try to resolve the issue with them." Sometimes they won't turn over the care because of the state of the finances. When this happens, I recommend that they consult with a financial manager to see if they can work out the money issues, so they don't have to be responsible for providing care.

Someone I know is in that situation and does what he can, but he's not the primary caregiver. He has siblings, so he keeps his part to a minimum. His relationship with his mom is such that they're not likely to ever resolve anything. He made the decision to do what he feels is his part, and his siblings take on the rest.

So that's another approach: share the care and limit how much contact you have if you're lucky enough to have other people who can help.

In another case, a daughter did not want to take her parents into her home. The parents had the means to stay in their home, and so the daughter was over there two or three times a day, supervising their in-home care. (She lived nearby and had the time available.) Those visits were enough to make her feel like her parents were well cared for, but she didn't have to be living in the same house with them, which would have taken a toll emotionally.

> 66
> Share the care and limit how much contact you have if you're lucky enough to have other people who can help.

MOURNING/GRIEVING

When your parents become elderly and require care, you might feel grief. Much of the mourning and the grieving that comes when caring for a parent often stems from a reversal of roles.

When you have role reversal, such as when you're caring for your parents, the traditional dynamic goes away. Many people feel as though they've lost their parent when this happens. When reality hits, you might go through a mourning process.

That happened to me. The first day my mother went in one of my own vans to one of my centers was devastating for me. I had brought my mother to live with me, and I decided that it would be good for her to be in one of my SarahCare adult day health centers, where my office was located. I wanted her to have some socialization, and I wanted her to have some time out of the house. Because she was in a wheelchair, to get her to the center, I had one of my vans come and pick her up. We got her dressed, took her down the ramp in the garage, and the driver, who I knew very well, put her on the wheelchair lift. And as the lift was going up, I started sobbing.

My husband asked, "What's wrong? She's going to *your* center in *your* building where *your* office is with *your* staff. You should be comfortable with that." And I said, "For the first time since my mother had this stroke, I realized she will never get better, and the mother I knew will never, ever come back." At that moment I realized it, and I had to go through a grieving process.

This sort of loss is similar to when you actually lose a parent. When that happens, I've heard people say, "I'm an orphan now. I'm all alone in the world." What they're really saying is "Even though I'm an independent, high-functioning person, in the back of my mind, I still felt as though I could depend on my mom or dad. They were my parent, and I still had that special relationship with them."

WHEN YOUR PARENT DOESN'T RECOGNIZE YOU

Another loss you might be grieving happens when a parent has dementia and doesn't recognize you. Sometimes it helps when families understand that their loved one's long-term memory is often still working. You might be aware of that but not understand the consequences.

The way it works is that the child your parent remembers (you) might be much, much younger. You're an adult now, and they don't recognize you because that part of their memory isn't working.

It's important for family members to understand what's going on because it makes that loss just a little bit easier.

A suggestion that might help them to know who you are: as you're walking into the room, start talking to them before you enter. Very often they'll recognize the voice even though they don't recognize the face.

Legal Decisions

If something happens to your parents, they might want you or a sibling to be responsible for certain aspects of their life. They might want to give you the right to write checks out of their account, for example, or make other legal decisions, whether or not they are incapacitated. Durable power of attorney (POA) gives you these rights.

Your parent can also designate someone to make decisions regarding their health should they become incapacitated. This is called a *healthcare proxy, medical power of attorney,* or *healthcare power of attorney.*

While the healthcare proxy and medical power of attorney forms—and instructions for what to do with them—can be found online, you can also fill these out using an estate attorney. You can use the same attorney to execute the durable power of attorney paperwork. They can explain all the rights and responsibilities that go with these powers and establish the powers in a way that works for your family. While lawyers can be costly, it is possible to find a lawyer who will prepare these papers—including a will—for a flat fee, if your estate is not terribly complicated.

Parents must think through who they are giving power to. I tell parents to discuss with their adult children ahead of time who gets which powers and why they've divided it that way. When children find out after the fact, they often put their own interpretation on it, and it can result in conflict.

There are various reasons why parents designate one child for specific roles. It is helpful to have the adult child who is the primary caregiver to have these POAs. We often experience situations in which the POA lives across the country and doesn't really see the condition of their parent and yet dictates care solutions. This results in frustration for the primary family caregiver who lives close by.

We have many situations in SarahCare where the primary caregiver is taking care of the parent, who's living in their home, and the caregiver doesn't have the durable power of attorney. They might want to send them to day care, or they might want home care, and the person who has durable power of attorney, who lives far away, is saying, "I don't think that's necessary. I talked to Mom on the phone, and she sounds fine to me. Why do you need any assistance or respite?"

Similar issues arise if you're in the middle of a healthcare crisis, a decision must be made, and the person who has the healthcare rights is living somewhere else. That can create tremendous problems.

Another reason for discussing it ahead of time is to prevent hurt feelings. My mother gave healthcare power of attorney to me instead of my brother. I asked her to discuss this with him ahead of time, and she didn't. He found out that I had healthcare power of attorney when she had her stroke and was very ill in the hospital. He was devastated.

The reason she did that was because my brother is a physician, and she didn't want him to have the responsibility for making medical decisions. She felt it would be a burden to him. He interpreted it completely differently and was very hurt.

I tell parents that they should be having these discussions ahead of time so that everybody knows what their thinking is and why they're doing what they're doing. That leaves matters open to discussion, and you might find that the decision you're about to make isn't the best one.

Finances

Whether or not your parents need you to step into the role of caregiver, as your parents age, it's a good idea to talk about financial issues.

If one parent has passed and your other parent is living alone, at least one person in your family should have a handle on your parent's monthly bills and where their assets are kept. I know someone whose father sent his children a spreadsheet monthly of the bills and when they needed to be paid. He was still paying his own bills, but if anything happened to him, his children could step in and take care of them if he was unable. Note that, if bills are paid online, someone should have access to passwords.

You might think it's not a great idea to take the finances out of your parent's hands. My mother was living independently and functioning fine when she said to me, "I'd like you to take care of my finances." I told her "no" because I wanted her to stay as sharp as possible. I didn't want her to give that up.

Looking back on it, I should have asked her more questions about why she wanted me to take it over and really get to the bottom of it. I realize now that she knew she was starting to decline. And it was a good idea for one of her children to have a hand in her finances.

> ### 💡 TIP: HOW ELDER SERVICES CAN HELP
>
> If you're not living near your parent, and they are having difficulties with the responsibility of paying their bills, look into elder services that are local to your parent. Many elder services agencies offer volunteers who can come and help with this.

Family Meetings

Family meetings to discuss a parent can sometimes be difficult, depending on the dynamics with your siblings. A little planning can smooth the way.

NEUTRAL THIRD PARTIES

If you think there's going to be a lot of disagreement and conflict at your family meeting, I recommend bringing in a third party who's neutral. You might need to bring in a professional so it's not you who's telling the family what you think needs to be done. Your siblings might question your motives and say things like, "You want to do it that way because of money" or "You're harboring resentment and want to put Dad away!" Involving a neutral third party who's a professional can defuse this sort of tension.

Some examples of a third party include a geriatric care manager (discussed in more detail in chapter 8) who has done an assessment or a physical therapist who's been working with your parent. But it's not always a healthcare professional. It might be a financial manager, an estate attorney, or a tax attorney. Sometimes you need those people to tell you what's really involved in the decisions that are being made and the consequences. They'll know the laws, rules, requirements, and benefits in the state where your parent is living.

If you're meeting with your siblings on your own, how do you deal with a situation that needs a tiebreaker?

Sometimes you get to the point where you say, "We can't figure this out on our own so why don't we consult with an expert?" And you must agree as to who you're going to consult. Then you end the meeting and have the next meeting with the person who'll give you enough information to get through the tiebreaker.

But sometimes, even with all of that, you still have people in conflict and angry. And at some point, whoever has the durable power of attorney is going to have to bite the bullet and make the decision that they think is best.

HOW TO CONDUCT A FAMILY MEETING

I like family meetings to have structure. The structure makes a big difference.

- First, figure out where you're going to hold the meeting. I don't recommend holding it at someone's home, where there are no boundaries on behavior or decorum. If your parent is in a hospital or rehab, sometimes the facility will give you access to a lounge or other area where you can meet. A restaurant or other public place will do as well, where anger will likely be kept in check.
- Include a neutral third party, such as a geriatric care manager.
- Everyone should agree on an agenda. What are you going to talk about and in what order?
- At the beginning of the meeting, hand out the agenda. Use it to stay on track and make sure you cover what you intended to cover.

A neutral party in a neutral place with a specific agenda is key.

INVOLVING THE SIBLINGS' SPOUSES

In some families—especially when you hold family meetings or have a major decision to make—everyone's involved. But sometimes, a brother-in-law or sister-in-law can undermine the process. Or sometimes there are too many opinions when you allow the in-laws to be involved.

It's nice when the spouses care enough to want to help, but at some point, someone might have to say, "It's only going to be the adult children" and exclude the spouses.

On the other hand, I just got done working with a family in which one of the daughters-in-law is always in the family meetings. The mother lives in the same city as the daughter-in-law, who does a lot for her. She goes to all the doctors' appointments. She's at the assisted living a couple times a week. She has a lot of very valuable information that's needed, and so for that reason, she's included.

Other than a situation like that, I would recommend keeping things simple and excluding the spouses.

LINGERING RESENTMENT BETWEEN SIBLINGS

When a parent dies, sometimes there's resentment among the siblings about how things were handled when they were still alive. That's why it's helpful if parents can make decisions and document them ahead of time. For example, I know someone who, when she was moving to assisted living, went through her house with Post-it notes and wrote names on each object as to who was getting what.

But it's not always the possessions that are at issue. It's often how the situation was handled. Maybe the parent was put in a nursing home over the objection of one of the siblings. Sometimes these emotional issues carry over long after the parent is gone.

It's for this reason that nurses, geriatric social workers, and palliative care professionals are extremely helpful when these types of decisions need to be made. They're familiar with the pros and cons and often understand family dynamics.

In the end, if one sibling says to you, "You should take care of Mom in your home," I recommend that you give them choices. You can say, "We have two choices. Either I'm sending them to you, and you can take care of them in your home, which is fine with me. Or, somehow or other, we have to come up with enough money to pay for live-in, around-the-clock care because what you're asking for is not something I'm capable of doing. Which of these two choices would you prefer?"

Sibling relationships can be complex, highly emotional, and full of rivalry. Old conflicts are old conflicts, and if you always resented your sister or your brother for whatever reason, you're not going to get past it unless you're willing to give it up. These emotions often become heightened when there is disagreement about the care of a parent.

Sometimes when there's conflict between siblings, you have to say to yourself, "You know what? This is their problem, not mine. I have to do what I think is best for Mom and Dad, and I'm just going to have to live with whatever their reaction is because there's nothing I can do at this point."

It might take an act of will to move past your anger or hurt feelings. You can either hold onto it or you can say, "I'm not going to ever get satisfaction from this. I'm going to move past it." And once you've made that decision, don't look back, as it moves the focus away from your parent.

Alternatively, you could try to resolve your conflicts. You could say, "I wish we had a better relationship, but you are choosing to stay in something that you think happened twenty or thirty years ago when we were both essentially children. If you choose to stay back there and make yourself continually unhappy, then that's up to you. But I'd prefer that we move forward as the adults we are now. That would be in the best interest of our parents."

I like to suggest using those words about choosing and choice a lot in a variety of circumstances, from raising children to dealing with siblings. These words help you to make it clear that that is what they have chosen. They are then responsible for their choices—not you.

FORGIVENESS

When you think back on decisions that you have made that have not necessarily been the best decisions, think through why you made that decision and why you did what you did. The conclusion you will usually come to is that you made the best decision possible based on the information you had at that time.

That's probably the perspective that the person you are having issues with is coming from: they did not realize the negative consequences of what they were doing, and at that time, thought that was the best decision possible, even though it was a terrible decision and it hurt people around them. Their intent was not to hurt, but they made a decision that was a very bad decision.

Sometimes looking at it from the other person's perspective in this manner can help you to forgive them.

When the Parent Won't Move

Some people refuse to move out of their home for the simple reason that they don't want to. There's not much you can do when another location is safest for them, but they won't go there.

Complex issues are involved when people won't move. I recommend that someone drills down to find out what's really going on. That's why a geriatric care manager can be helpful; parents will often reveal things to them that they wouldn't necessarily tell their families.

Sometimes, when people refuse to move out of their homes, they are dealing with issues that might not be obvious. They might be overwhelmed with the idea of sorting through their possessions and packing up. In this case, certified senior move managers can help. They're primarily social workers and nurses, but their job is to come in and help to sort through things and give things away. They can also help to decide where to move to and figure out how much furniture they can bring with them. It can be hard for anyone to visualize their furniture and other possessions in a new space, and this can be a blocker that prevents your parent from moving.

A few years ago, I was invited to present at the Annual Conference of Senior Move Managers. To help them to understand what people experience when they move to much smaller quarters, such as assisted living, I asked each of them to go home that evening and pack everything that was important to them into two boxes. As you would expect, they returned the next day very frustrated and upset. But they began to understand what it means to have to put your entire life into a few boxes. This is a major reason why some people refuse to move. Discussions about giving away meaningful items to people while you are still alive, explaining to them what each object means to you and why you want them to have it is very helpful for moving this process forward.

Recently, I was talking with a woman whose family told me that she needs to go to an assisted living facility, and she was refusing to go. When I started to drill down with her about why she wasn't going, she said, "I need new clothes. I can't go to that assisted living in the clothes that I already have. I'm not comfortable." And I asked her, "If we got you new clothes, do you think you would be willing to move?" And she said, "Yeah, I would."

That's not the first time I've heard this.

In addition to worrying about clothing and furniture, your parent might also be concerned about the caregiver who's been working in their home. They might tell you, "The caregiver that's in my home has told me that if she loses this job, she won't be able to get another one. And she's a single mom." Once you understand their reason for hesitating, it's easier to arrive at solutions.

STAYING SAFE AT HOME

If your elderly parent won't go to a safer environment, insist that they get a Lifeline or similar device and that they have it with them wherever they are in the house. Consider whether a stairlift, shower railings, and other safety devices are appropriate as well and help them to get them installed.

Grandchildren

As a parent, helping to form relationships between your children and your parents can give your child a life skill for dealing with older people. Spending time with a grandparent who has hearing loss, uses a walker, is a fall risk, is ill, or maybe even has dementia is a learning experience for your children. They will take that with them for their entire lives, and it will inform how they relate to people and eventually with their own parents—you!

HOW THEY MIGHT BE FEELING

Children understand what's going on. Give them an opportunity to ask questions, especially when someone has dementia. It can be very difficult for the children in that situation because the grandparents might look the same physically. It's not like when they're ill, and they look different.

Kids can pick up on the fact that there's something going on medically, even if you don't tell them explicitly. Don't underestimate that children see that things are changing in the family. They are apt to have a lot of questions,

> 66
> Don't underestimate that children see that things are changing in the family.

and you need to sit with them and talk to them about it. There are also plenty of excellent books available for explaining this kind of thing to children. You can search the internet for "books for teaching about sick grandparents" to find a plethora of results and select some that suit your circumstances.

And children, depending on their age, often have other concerns. "This is my grandmother, so she's old," they might think. "That's fine. But what about my mom? Will she be like this when she's older?" Issues of life cycle and death sometimes appear for children that you might need to discuss.

VISITING WITH GRANDPARENTS

If your parents move to an assisted living facility or nursing home, at some point, you'll probably bring your children to visit them. You'll need to talk to your children about their comfort level and prepare them for what's going to happen there. And you need to have a plan for the time you'll spend there with them.

I don't recommend bringing children into a setting where you expect them to sit in a chair and listen to an adult conversation. I know someone who used to bring a ball with them, and the children would just toss the ball back and forth while they were visiting. It worked to keep them distracted. Someone else brought a book because her mother used to love to read to the children. She could still do that even though she had had a stroke. Someone had to turn the pages for her, but she could still read to the children and share that bond.

If your children are teenagers, you have to decide: Are you going to let them have their phones while they're there and they can do whatever they want to do? Are you going to allow them to wear their earbuds? There's no right or wrong answer—you just have to think these situations through ahead of time and communicate the plan to them.

Sometimes facilities such as nursing homes have snacks available (like milk and cookies), or you can bring a special treat when you visit. And that becomes a pleasant part of the ritual for when you visit Grandma or Grandpa.

The same issues arise when visiting aging parents in their homes. The kids have to have something to do, and you have to think through ahead of time what they can and can't do and what you're comfortable with. Sometimes there are compromises. "We're going to have tea in the afternoon, and during tea you can't have your phone, and you can't have your earbuds in. But the rest of the time, it's fine." That's a perfectly good agreement.

When a Child Is Ill

Care issues for our spouse or partner and parents are bound to happen as they age. But children, too, can be born with or develop issues that require you to have skills that fall outside the usual parenting path. We'll look at those in the next chapter. ❧

CHAPTER 7

Children with Special Needs

In the first several chapters of this book, I talked about taking care of children, from infancy to adulthood. Raising your children and dealing with all the care issues involved can be all encompassing. But what if your child develops a health issue or has special needs that require additional care?

Family Matters

When a child has special needs, whether it's a health issue or a developmental one, their care can take up an enormous amount of time and energy. It can be exhausting. Your whole focus is on that child because he or she needs a lot of your attention.

In these situations, if you aren't intentional about keeping your other relationships on track, you might start running into problems. Marriages can end in divorce, or your other children might become angry and estranged because of all the focus and time that's spent on the child who has a special need.

How can you avoid these problems? Sometimes you have to do what's difficult, which is to bring in someone else to help. Usually it's a family member—your siblings or your parents—or it can be a close family friend. Whoever it is, I strongly recommend using that help to maintain some balance in your family.

YOUR OTHER CHILDREN

Family members might offer to come in and help. They might offer to spend time with your other children and give them attention. If you can't be home because, say, you're staying at the hospital with your ill child, focused time with another family member can certainly be helpful to your other children.

I generally recommend, though, that the helper spend their time with the child with special needs, if possible. This approach allows you to spend time with your other children. It also gives your child with special needs the opportunity to interact with someone other than you.

If you're not at home, though, and this isn't possible, think about how you can let your child who is at home know that you love them and care about them. I know someone who was in the hospital with her ill child for two weeks at a time. She recorded herself reading a book to her other child, complete with chimes so he knew when to turn the page. With today's technology, you can FaceTime, send voice recordings, make a video, and use many other means to "be there"—virtually, at least.

I know another family that has two children, the younger of whom is on the autism spectrum and requires full-time care. It's hard for the parents to give attention to their child who is developing normally. They were fortunate to have a niece who was skilled and could come and take care of their child with autism. This allowed them to take their other son on an occasional family vacation, even if for a few days. They were able to give him these types of experiences because they allowed family members to develop a close relationship with their child with special needs and care for him.

FOCUS ON YOUR MARRIAGE

When your child has issues beyond the regular day-in, day-out needs that come with childhood, you have to give extra attention to your marriage. Perhaps you are sharing the load when it comes to caring for your child, or perhaps it's all on one parent. In either case, you'll need to squeeze in time as a couple if you want to keep your marriage healthy.

There's a line from the movie *My Big Fat Greek Wedding 2*, in which the couple, who at this point are parents, are planning to go out to dinner. As they're getting ready, an aunt says to the wife, "Remember, you were a girlfriend before you were a mother." After that conversation, much to her husband's surprise, she gets all dolled up for dinner.

That scene always stuck with me. Sometimes it helps to remind yourself about the importance of your relationship with your partner and put forth extra effort to show you care.

When I was taking care of my mother, I managed to go away with my husband. It made me really nervous to do so, and it wasn't for more than one or two nights, but we went away.

Even though I was anxious about it, it was very good for me. First of all, it gave me a chance to sleep, which was really important. And second, it gave my husband and me some time to be together without all the stress of what was going on.

It's the same when your child needs special care.

Whether you take a short break, enjoy an hour's walk in the park, or meet for a lunch date, it doesn't matter. The point is you need to say, "Making time for my marriage is important to me. And it is important to my spouse." And then you need to go ahead and take action.

SELF-CARE

If you're your child's main caregiver, you're probably thinking about everyone but yourself. To be able to take care of another person, you need to keep yourself healthy, both physically and emotionally. Understandably, the latter can be difficult when you are worrying about your child. But do take the time to get yourself out and do something pleasurable. It could be for some time with a friend. Maybe you can even enjoy a nice, long phone call while sitting on your porch. If you're with your child in the hospital, maybe you can just sit in the lounge by yourself or step outside for some fresh air while a child-life specialist spends time with your child. Have your child participate in whatever organized activities there might be on the unit, if they're able.

You can't do everything. Just do one thing for yourself this week.

Maybe you've not gone to your book club for six months, and you finally say, "This is ridiculous. I'm going to book club." Or you decide to participate in whatever your passion is that you've been missing out on. The point is you have to start doing at least one thing for yourself.

At the end of my radio show, sometimes I'll say, "You can't do everything. Just do one thing for yourself this week. Even if it's for five or ten minutes, do one thing for yourself." It could be something as slight as giving yourself an extra ten minutes in the shower. Whatever it is, just do it!

Concerns about the Future

When you have a child with special needs—someone who can't live independently—the situation creates worry. "What's going to happen later?" you wonder. I hear that a lot.

What I usually say to parents is "I understand that you're very fearful, and it's a very scary situation." When anyone is dependent on you for their care, you need a plan B. That's especially true when you have a child with special needs.

WHERE WILL THEY LIVE?

My friends' oldest child was in a bad bicycle/car accident. He had permanent brain damage. As parents, they were getting more and more anxious and more and more fearful because this child was living with them at home. They had built a new home with ramps and a roll-in shower. It had everything for him that he needed. But they were getting older. What if one of them suddenly had a health crisis? What would happen then?

They ended up making the decision to move him into a residential setting during the week. He came home on the weekends, and it ended up working really well. The residential setting gave him some socialization, and he was with other people his age, working at his functional level throughout the week. He came home on the weekends and on the holidays.

Eventually, they did hit a healthcare crisis. They would not have been able to continue to take care of him at that point. But he had already transitioned into the residential setting, so it didn't turn out to be such a crisis.

With spouses and parents, people say, "I'm really afraid. What if I'm not here? What if I can't function?" It's the same thing with children. You need to try to make plans for where they're going to be, what they're going to do, and you need to start that planning early. Realize, though, that your plans might change because the child's ability to function can change.

HOW WILL THEY BE SUPPORTED FINANCIALLY?

You also need to plan financially for when you're not there. Who's going to take care of the child, and how will it get paid for?

I'm working with two families in which the other children help to take care of their sibling with special needs. That's great and fine now, but they come and go as they please. What's going to happen when the parents aren't there anymore, or the parents are incapacitated or not able to be the primary caregivers? Are the children still going to be able to come and go as they please? When we sat down at a family meeting, they realized the answer was no. So where is he going to live? Who's going to live in the home around the clock? And who's going to pay for all of that? Everyone was looking at each other around the table without an answer.

We finally got to a plan for how we were going to work that out. But if I hadn't called that family meeting and something happened, they would have been in crisis. And then everyone would have been scurrying.

One helpful resource for addressing these issues is an estate attorney. Very often, the lawyers who specialize in estate planning deal with families who have young children or adult children with special needs. They often have suggestions you might not have thought of. They're very good at setting up trusts and helping you to make arrangements for the future. ❧

CHAPTER 8

Common Issues for Providing Healthcare

Taking care of a child, spouse, partner, or a parent each comes with its own set of issues, which I'll discuss in the chapters that follow. However, many issues are common to any situation in which your loved one is experiencing a health issue.

Employment Issues

When a family member becomes ill, and you need to care for them, it can create issues at work. In fact, caregiving for family members (called *informal caregiving* because you're not getting paid for it) costs

$522 billion a year in the United States, according to the RAND Corporation.[4]

TELLING YOUR MANAGER

 TIP: TALKING TO YOUR BOSS

Write down what you mean to say ahead of time—even if it's bullet points—and bring your "cheat sheet" with you.

When a family member's health issue will affect your work, you'll need to tell your supervisor or manager what's going on and explain your needs. That conversation should follow the same guidelines as for any negotiation.

First, state the problem simply, in just a few sentences. It's not necessary or helpful for your manager to know the full nature of the health condition, how it came about, and what's involved in the care. You might feel comfortable saying that your parent had a stroke or that your partner is undergoing chemotherapy, and that's okay if you want to do so.

But you don't need to provide any details at all. In fact, you can keep it as simple as, "We had a family health crisis that I'll need to attend to over the next several weeks" or "My child has a chronic health condition that will affect my work hours on an ongoing basis." That level of detail is fine. Too much information might even discour-

---

4   "Cost of Informal Caregiving for U.S. Elderly Is $522 Billion Annually," rand.org (RAND Corporation, October 27, 2014), https://www.rand.org/news/press/2014/10/27. html#:~:text=Cost%20of%20Informal%20Caregiving%20for%20U.S.%20Elderly%20 Is%20%24522%20Billion%20Annually,-For%20Release&text=The%20price%20 tag%20for%20informal,a%20new%20RAND%20Corporation%20study.

age your manager from accommodating you if what you're describing sounds overwhelming.

Next, state very clearly what you need. Do you need to come in later and stay later? Work remotely? Reduce your hours? Whatever you need, be clear and succinct about it. Tell them

- What you can do.

- What you can't do.

- The time period involved.

It's possible that you'll need to ask to modify your responsibilities. Sometimes people in this situation decline a promotion or take on a lesser role. Those are options to think through before you approach your boss. State the problem, what you need, and your proposed solution. The conversation might go something like this.

I've been traveling every other week. I can't continue to do that anymore; I need to be based at home. But here's how I can manage it.

DEALING WITH YOUR COWORKERS

Another work issue involves your relationships with your colleagues. Very often what happens when you're dealing with a family health crisis is that you'll start taking calls from home in the middle of the day from home healthcare workers or family members. When you begin taking non-work-related calls frequently, it can impact your colleagues. At first, they'll feel sympathetic toward you. After a while, though, they might find that they're covering for you, so it affects them.

For this reason, how care is delivered when you're not there is important to settle on. You need to let home healthcare workers know that they have to call you in a real emergency, but otherwise you need to schedule the times that you're going to connect throughout the day. You can say, "I will call you at 11:30. Please hold your questions until then, and then I will call you again at 2:30." Use a schedule that works for you.

If the constant calls are coming from your parent or your spouse, then you need to think about either getting a caregiver in your home or sending them to an adult day health center during the day so you can put a stop to the calls. Otherwise, you won't be able to function in your job.

Once you have made these arrangements, communicate with your colleagues frequently enough so they understand what's going on and what you're trying to do. They will appreciate your efforts to reduce the interruptions and perform your job duties.

DEALING WITH DIRECT REPORTS

Having caregiving responsibilities can also affect the people who are working for you. Suddenly, you're not as available to them. They don't know what's going on. They might misinterpret lack of communication that they're in trouble. It's easier on them if you disclose to them that you have a family healthcare crisis going on, and you're resolving it as quickly as possible.

Remember, too, that however you're handling your healthcare crisis with your family, whatever you're doing for yourself needs to be done for them should they find themselves in a similar situation. Otherwise, they become resentful. Their thinking might be something like, "My boss has a personal healthcare crisis. Suddenly, she's not coming in every morning until ten o'clock. But when I ask to come in late because of my kid's health problem, she tells me no."

Monitor your behavior very carefully to make sure you are being fair.

BEING PRESENT AT WORK AND AT HOME ... VIRTUALLY

Nowadays, depending on the type of work you do, there are options for being able to provide care while also working. For example, many of us have become very comfortable performing our jobs at home and conducting business over Zoom, Skype, Slack, and the many other tools that facilitate virtual communication.

On top of that, doctors' appointments can be done through tele-health. And very often, if you ask, they can add you to a telehealth or in-person visit from your workplace. In other words, someone else can take your parent or spouse to the appointment, or, if they're doing it by teletherapy, you can be included. This technique can reduce your time away from your work desk.

IF YOU HAVE TO LEAVE YOUR JOB

What if you feel you need to leave the job? It happens. While it can free you to provide the needed care, it can be a big strain financially.

If your spouse is disabled, they might be getting disability payments from their employer or from Social Security, and that can help. Also, in some states, a program exists in which family caregivers, after a short period of training, can get paid for taking care of their family member. Unfortunately, this program goes by different names in every state since it's not a federal program. To find out if your state has such a program, call your local Medicaid office or your area agencies on aging. They will be familiar with whether these programs exist and how to access them.

If you find a way to get paid to give care, make sure your other family members know about it. For a relative such as an aunt, uncle, parent, or grandparent, I recommend that you write up a one-page agreement between you and the family member you'll be caring for. The agreement should state what you're going to do and how much you'll get paid. Make sure that everyone in your family who might have a financial interest knows about it. This protects you from being accused later on of taking financial advantage of your loved one.

I went through this with a family in which a niece had been very attentive to her aunt in the hospital and then in rehab. When the aunt was ready to go home, her immediate family wanted a paid caregiver, so they planned to approach the niece and offer to pay her.

Out of nowhere, a cousin showed up and offered to step in and take care of the aunt. When the aunt was hospitalized, this cousin hadn't even called to see how she was doing. When there was money involved, suddenly she appeared.

Politics like this are not uncommon in families, which is why it's important to put matters involving money in writing.

A HELPFUL RESOURCE

Family Caregiver Alliance has done a lot of research on the topic of caregiving and employment. They've written on the impact on businesses and on caregivers. Their website is caregiver.org, and I recommend that you visit it to explore the resources they offer.

Feeling Squeamish

You might be providing healthcare for the first time in your life. And it may be difficult to talk about, but you might feel squeamish or even disgusted by what you have to do. If you're not used to dealing with urinary issues, incontinency, blood, or giving injections, it might be a major problem for you in providing care.

If you can't get past that feeling, you'll have to get somebody else to handle what you can't because you can't give that negative message to the person you're caring for. I know someone whose son had daily home infusions, and she was nervous to administer them. "What if I make a mistake?" she said. It's scary.

Sometimes you have to work through it. But sometimes you have to find another way. Maybe a visiting nurse can come, which might even be covered by insurance. If it's a long-term need, you'll have to either find someone else to provide the care or work through your fears. You could even ask a neighbor to come by on a regular basis if you have a strong relationship with them. It doesn't necessarily have to be a family member. It just needs to be somebody who can get to your house frequently enough and who can be trained to perform the procedure.

> **66**
> If you're too squeamish to do something, you need to be honest about it.

If you're too squeamish to do something, you need to be honest about it. I had a friend whose husband needed wound care. The wound-care nurse visited two or three times a week. But the bandage needed to be changed and the wound cleaned twice a day, so my friend was supposed to do it the rest of the time. But when she started to do it, she'd have to go into the bathroom and vomit.

I said to her, "You've got to tell the nurse what's going on, and you've got to have her help you find a way to handle this. Because what's happening is you're not changing the dressing, and it's becoming a problem. You need to be honest about this. It's okay. Not everyone can do this."

I had another friend who was providing care to her husband. She called me one morning and said, "I just cannot do this. I don't know what to do."

Because I have access to nurses, I got hold of one who had retired, and I said, "Are you willing to come into this home twice a day? They'll pay you." Sometimes retired nurses are more than willing to do this in a short-term situation. They might not want to do this every day for the rest of their life. But they might do it every day for two weeks or three weeks.

Whatever solution you land on, you need to find a way to provide the needed care.

Venting Your Frustrations

Frustration is very common when providing care. There are various levels of frustration. Sometimes, the frustration is with the insurance company. Sometimes, it's with the medical professionals when you're sitting by the phone waiting for a response. But sometimes it's that things are not happening the way you want them to or as you thought they were going to. Or they're not going as quickly as you expected, and you're generally frustrated.

Usually when I'm dealing with people who are that frustrated, I tell them they need to be in a support group, or they need to be seeing someone privately. Or they need a really good friend who's willing to go out and get either a hot chocolate or a drink because they need to vent. Because unless you can find a solution to this frustration, which usually isn't readily available, the only way you're going to be able to get through it is to talk it through.

Know that frustration comes with the territory. It might feel like you're alone and that everyone else is functioning better than you are.

But the fact is that what you're experiencing, while unique to you, is something that everybody comes up against in one form or another. You are not alone.

Dealing with Professionals in the Healthcare World

Navigating the medical world can be overwhelming, whether at an appointment or in the hospital. While you will come to know the professionals you are working with and how to get what you need from them, common situations do arise.

COMMUNICATIONS

The number one issue in dealing with professionals is how to get the information you need and the answers you want. If you don't like the answer that you're getting, you need to ask more questions. It's your right to say to a professional, "Wait a minute. I still have more questions, and I really need some answers." It's also your right to get a second opinion.

> To facilitate communication when visiting with a medical professional, always write down your questions ahead of time because you're likely to forget once you are face to face.

To facilitate communication when visiting with a medical professional, always write down your questions ahead of time because you're likely to forget once you are face to face. Sometimes I advise people to bring a friend with them because sometimes the friend who's not emotionally involved can listen more carefully and ask questions you might not have thought to ask.

WHO ARE YOUR PROVIDERS?

There are many kinds of providers out there. What's the difference between a nurse practitioner and a physician's assistant? What care can they provide and not provide? You might need to become familiar with the difference between palliative care and hospice. Both provide comfort care, but with hospice, there's no intention to cure the patient. With palliative care, there may or may not be.

It's a real educational process, but it's worthwhile to go online, do some research, and begin to become familiar with the vocabulary and what it means to you and your family member.

INSURANCE

Insurance can be difficult to navigate. For example, you might get a bill that you don't understand or be charged for something that you think should be covered.

While insurance policies can be hard to parse, if you are in a situation where you are responsible for getting coverage, it pays to understand the policy. Read the policy description, and if you have any questions, call the insurance company's Customer Service number to get clarification. Understanding how your deductible works and what is and is not covered will help you to make decisions or to deal with a billing error.

And billing errors happen often. How do you deal with that? I know someone whose son was in the hospital in a room overnight. The insurance company billed for an emergency room visit rather than covering the event as a hospital admission, which provided more coverage. She had to argue the point repeatedly that her son was in a room on the floor. Despite significant resistance, she eventually got the claim covered in full.

In these circumstances, you have to understand your coverage, be persistent, and ask to speak to a supervisor at the insurance company if you're not getting the answer you believe is correct or an explanation that makes sense.

Another insurance issue that arises has to do with long-term care insurance. People often assume that long-term care insurance, if they have it, is only for nursing homes. That's not accurate. If you do have long-term care insurance, talk to your broker to find out what it actually covers because very often, it covers home care, and sometimes it covers adult day health centers.

REHAB PLACEMENT

When a rehab placement is recommended, you have to ask questions of the social workers and the discharge planners. If you're uncomfortable with the advice you're getting—if they're telling you to go to this rehab center or that hospice—visit the facility yourself. Go see where your family member is going before they actually go, and make sure it's where you want them to be.

There are different kinds of rehab centers. Some inpatient rehab centers are very intensive. To qualify for placement there, you have to be able to do therapy for three hours a day. These tend to be very high quality. A rehab center that's in a nursing home, on the other hand, only has to provide therapy one hour a day, and they might not be as good as inpatient rehab facilities. That's why I recommend that you ask questions and visit these facilities ahead of time.

You might like a facility and find you can't get your family member in. There might not be a bed, or there might be some other issue that would prevent them from taking your family member. For that reason, it's good to find several options that would satisfy you.

On the other hand, if you are told no, you can still try to see if it's possible. Because you might be told "no" by one person, but there might be a way to make it happen. Talk to the people both at the hospital and at the facility you want to go to, and make sure you understand the obstacles to see if there might be a way around them.

I also recommend that you talk to your family member. I was able to get Frank into the rehab center I wanted because I would talk to him. I would go in the morning and say to him, "The physical therapist is coming in. If you're not cooperative, you're going to end up in the rehab in the nursing home. I don't think that's what you want, so shake a leg and get moving. I know it's hard, but you've got to do it because, otherwise, we're going to have no choice of where you can go." That served as a reminder to him that there was a lot at stake and that he needed to work hard and cooperate.

OTHER PLACEMENT OPTIONS

If you're trying to figure out whether an older family member should go home with a home health aide or to a nursing home, I have found that getting a neutral third party involved works best. I suggest people hire a certified geriatric care manager if they can or go to the area agency on aging in their area. Have someone do a professional assessment, which they then can discuss with the family.

GERIATRIC CARE MANAGERS

If you're looking for advice on how to get the most appropriate care for your spouse or parent, I recommend that you find a certified geriatric care manager to serve as your consultant. You can find certified geriatric care managers online.

You pay certified geriatric care managers directly for their services. These services can be costly, but the advantage is that these care managers are neutral. They are not paid for placements.

If you can't afford a certified geriatric care manager, then the area agencies on aging in every state have nurses who can come in, do an assessment, and recommend services and programs.

Some organizations offer consultants who are paid by a facility for every patient they recommend who is placed. I find that these consultants tend to recommend nursing homes over anything else. The second most likely recommendation is an assisted living facility. Nursing homes and assisted living facilities that pay them will tend to get more referrals. Home and community-based services are referred much less often because they don't get as much money for that referral.

Recently, I performed one of these assessments for an older parent. After spending time with the patient, I was able to talk to all the children at the same time and say, "Here's my assessment, and here are the recommendations that I'm making to you based on it." It wasn't coming from the son who was the primary caregiver; it was coming from an outside source. Getting an objective opinion removed the family dynamics from the decision-making process and allowed them to move forward with less conflict.

Monitoring Care in the Hospital

When your loved one is in the hospital, you might not be able to be there around the clock. However, understanding the rhythms of hospital life can help you to be there at the right times to ensure they are getting the care they need so you can stay on top of what's happening.

WHAT TIME ARE MEDICATIONS ADMINISTERED?

One thing to know is when your family member is supposed to get their medications so you can monitor whether they are getting them. If you can be on premises when the medications are administered, that can help. Some medications need to be delivered within a specific timeframe. Sometimes an hour delay is okay, but sometimes it's not. Understanding when the medications need to be delivered and seeing that they are administered can ensure the patient's safety.

For example, I know someone whose child was receiving chemotherapy. Within an hour after the chemotherapy, the child was supposed to get a particular infusion. The timing was critical. The mom found that not only was the nurse not there on time, but the medication was administered incorrectly. She had to alert a nurse to get the infusion going and then call the nurse again when she noticed the error.

You need to stay on top of the care needs in the hospital. This is one of the tougher aspects of caregiving for a family member. Did they have the procedure that was planned? Unfortunately, mistakes do happen, so you need to be the advocate.

WHEN DOCTORS ARE ROUNDING/ SHIFT CHANGES

It can be helpful to know when the doctors are rounding. When the doctors are in the room, it might be the only time you can get your questions answered by the key people involved in your family member's care. If you miss the team, you might be able to get a resident or attendant to answer questions, or you might need to ask a nurse. But you might not get as full a picture as you would have if you had been there yourself.

Sometimes doctors don't always round at a set time, and the team might not round at all on the weekends. But you can always find out when nurses are doing their change of shifts so you can be there when the new nurse comes on. I like to be there at the change of shifts because I want to make sure I can tell the nurse who's coming on board anything I might need for them to know.

 TIP:

For the times when you are away from the hospital, make sure you know who at the hospital you can call if you need to know what's going on and the best way to get hold of them. And they, of course, need to know how to get ahold of you!

TAKING CONTROL

If your family member is admitted at a teaching hospital, they might have a condition that's of interest to a physician and their students when they are rounding. Or a medical student on the floor might ask a lot of questions out of interest. If you and the patient are exhausted, and the patient is being used as a teaching tool, it's okay in those circumstances to advocate—for both of you. Let the team know that you need sleep, and they should come back later. It's important that students have hands-on learning experiences at teaching hospitals, but it shouldn't be at the expense of the patient's comfort.

KEEPING YOUR FAMILY MEMBER'S PHYSICIAN INVOLVED

The hospital might tell you that only the hospitalist is allowed to see your family member. If you've had a physician who has taken care of your family member for a long period of time, that physician knows the patient's history and should know that their patient is in the hospital. So, I recommend that you at least call the office and let them know that your family member is in the hospital (or send an email if you communicate with the physician that way) because, very often, the hospital won't do it.

Learning to Cope with Providing Care at Home

One of the most difficult things to deal with when a family member is ill or recovering from hospitalization is being the one who provides the care. Your family member is coming home from a hospital or rehab center, and suddenly you find the staff throwing information at you, like a set of instructions or a list of medications. Or they might be telling you about something more complicated, like how to transfer them from the bed to a wheelchair or how to help in the bathroom.

All of these needs can quickly become overwhelming,

GETTING READY FOR DISCHARGE

I recommend that, as soon as your family member goes into the hospital or into rehab, you start the discussion about how to prepare for what's going to happen when they are discharged, such as the equipment and materials you will need.

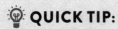 **QUICK TIP:**

Start planning for discharge at the beginning of the hospitalization or rehab, not at discharge. That will give you time to get the equipment you need or make any modifications to your home.

If you're going to need railings or ramps installed, they'll likely tell you the day before discharge, which is unhelpful. You need to start that conversation from day one or day two. Ask the physical therapist or occupational therapist: What do you think we're going to need? What equipment do I need for bathing? Whom do I contact to get this equipment installed? What companies do you recommend?

PROVIDING CARE

The first time Frank came home from the hospital, he was on fourteen medications. Even though I'm in healthcare, I had never managed medications. Suddenly I had six pages of instructions detailing which medications were taken when. I had to make an Excel sheet to get it all organized.

Then a friend told me about prefilled daily pill packs. A variety of companies provide this service. Ask your pharmacist or your insurance company about how to obtain medications this way.

I also recommend that, when a healthcare professional is demonstrating how to do something, take a video of it. When the physical therapist showed me how to help Frank get out of bed, I took a video so I could look at it and remind myself how to do it.

As for bathing an adult patient, it's possible that you can find an adult day health center that will take care of showering. At our SarahCare centers, we have roll-in showers, so we can handle bathing for families that can't handle it at home. Even if a home healthcare aide comes to your house, it might be difficult for them to get them into the shower. In that case, you might want to look into adult day health centers to see if they offer this service.

> When a healthcare professional is demonstrating how to do something, you take a video of it.

THREE KEY STEPS TO LEARNING A NEW MEDICAL PROCEDURE

The professionals you're dealing with might have their own way of teaching. But take control of the situation. Tell them:

1. Talk me through what we're going to do.
2. Next, show me how to do it.
3. Most importantly, have me do it one time in front of you. I have to show you that I know how to do this so that when I get my family member home, I'm comfortable with the procedure.

The first time you do something—whether it's flushing a feeding tube or changing a dressing—you don't want to be at home by yourself, where you might be flustered and forget the instructions.

SCOPING OUT PUBLIC PLACES

When I was taking care of my mother when she was in a wheelchair, I called a restaurant and asked whether they were handicapped accessible. They told me they were. But when I showed up, there were two steps going up to the entrance and no ramp.

That wasn't the first or last time that happened. Whenever you are bringing someone who has mobility challenges to a public place, you need to check out the situation in advance. Sometimes a phone call might be the best you can do, but as my experience with the restaurant showed, that doesn't always work. If that's your only option, ask questions that are as specific as possible. For example, for sporting events, find out where the seats are that accommodate wheelchairs. Do the same for movie theaters because often these seats are too close, and it's hard on everyone's neck to see the screen.

While getting your questions answered can be helpful, if you can, go to these places ahead of time and see what it's really like.

If you're taking your partner to the hospital for an appointment, usually a valet can take your car and provide you with a wheelchair. A wheelchair can be helpful even if the patient can walk. Sometimes the ramp can be quite long or it's a great distance from your car to the front entrance and then to the elevator.

Call, or check the hospital website before you go to understand where to go for valet service.

If you need to travel by airplane, you should also arrange for a wheelchair in advance for the same reasons. Furthermore, if your partner can't walk down the aisle of the airplane to your seats, you might need a special type of wheelchair for that purpose. Again, contact the airport or the airline. Their websites will have information on how to go about this.

When you're traveling, also consider looking into renting an electric scooter. Some hotels have wheelchairs with extra-large wheels that you can use for going to the beach. Be assertive about what you want. Call, tell them what you are trying to do, and ask if they can you get what you need to make it happen.

A lot of accommodations are available in the US, such as tour guides who can address mobility issues. There are also car services, such as Curb, that offer handicapped-accessible vehicles.

If you're caring for someone with mobility issues or another disability, you don't need to feel like you're in prison. Life doesn't have to end because of a physical problem. It just might take a little time and effort—and probably money—to make it happen.

Taking Care of Yourself

If you're taking care of another person, you need to take care of yourself. When you don't have physical or mental energy, you're likely to have difficulties handling the responsibilities that come with being a caregiver. If you're tired or hungry, you might find that you have less control over your emotions. You might become tearful or anxious.

I can't stress enough how fundamental quality sleep is to your well-being. You might be tempted to stay up overnight to tend to your spouse, but I can tell you from personal experience that it's not healthy for you, and it doesn't help you to provide better care.

In my situation, even though I had caregivers for Frank, I was sleeping in the same room with him. That guaranteed a poor night's sleep for me due to the equipment in his room and the care he required. But I wanted to be there if the caregivers needed my help or if they stepped away and something unexpected happened.

In reality, my help was needed at times. Sometimes I helped with the logistics, and sometimes my mere presence was needed to keep his anxiety down. Even when he was in the hospital and I was at home, one of the nurses on the overnight shift called me in because they needed me to keep him calm. They told me, "The minute you walk in the room, it's like air being released from a balloon. All the tension dissipates, and he calms down immediately."

So, to a degree, the sleep interruption was unavoidable. But, in retrospect I should have slept some nights in another bedroom. The caregivers were right there. They were good. Once I got to trust them, I should have gone to another bedroom and slept.

At one point when Frank was in the hospital, I was there around the clock. Finally, one of his physicians came in and said, "It's ten o'clock at night. You're here, and you look horrible. You're going to get sick. I'm going to get a sitter in here from 11:00 p.m. to 7:00 a.m., and you're going to go home."

I hadn't even known that a sitter was a possibility. If you're in a similar situation, talk to the hospital staff about strategies for getting the care your family member needs during the overnight shifts so you can sleep. And if you have offers of help from friends and family, don't hesitate to use that time to sleep.

Durable Medical Equipment

Durable medical equipment (DME) includes items such as wheelchairs, walkers, canes, and beds. You might encounter two issues regarding DME: getting the right equipment and getting it paid for by insurance.

GETTING THE RIGHT EQUIPMENT

People come into our centers all the time with the wrong equipment because they bought it off the shelf. My suggestion is that you visit a store that specializes in selling DME with someone that's knowledgeable about and trained in medical equipment.

One place to get help is from the person who is recommending the equipment, like the physical therapist. Some small businesses also have employees who are specially trained to make recommendations.

GETTING REIMBURSED FOR DME

If you want to get reimbursed by insurance, then you need a prescription. That's why it's best to go through the rehab specialist, who can write the prescription and then order the equipment for you.

Alternatively, when you leave the hospital, very often the social workers will put in the prescriptions to a company they deal with, who will then deliver the equipment to you. Even so, you need to be on your toes and ask questions. For example, Medicare paid for a hospital bed for my husband, but I wondered whether the mattress would handle his weight. When I found out the type of mattress being supplied, I ordered a more appropriate mattress for him. I did have to pay some money out of pocket for that, but it was necessary for his comfort

In terms of navigating Medicare or the financial end, the social workers in the hospital can help you with that. The problem is that they're always overwhelmed because they carry too many cases. You need to be forceful about getting the answers you need while still being nice to them. (Always be nice to the hospital staff!) Try something like the following.

I need to talk to you about this equipment before we order it, and I really must insist on speaking to you about this. When do you have time today? I know you're very busy, but it's critical that I get your help with this.

Being Prepared for a Crisis

It's important that you have a crisis plan—what I call a plan B—in case something happens to you or there's a crisis involving the person you're caring for. Rather than dealing with a crisis in the moment, figure out how you will handle things ahead of time. Crisis-mode decisions rarely work out!

For example, suppose you're taking care of your spouse who is incapacitated. Suddenly, you're out in your icy driveway to get the mail, and you slip, fall, and break your leg. What's going to happen now? You're the primary caregiver. What's going to happen to the person you're caring for? Or suppose you have to take your parent to the hospital in an emergency. Who's going to walk your dog or meet your child at the bus?

You need a plan for those situations.

Another way to prepare for a crisis is to make sure your list of who you need to call, and their numbers are posted in your house as well as programmed into your phone. Because when you're in the middle of an urgent situation and you need to make a call, you can't always remember what to do.

I advise families to think through those kind of crisis plans, get those plan Bs in order, and make sure everybody's alerted. Then, make sure that it's all posted somewhere you can easily see it, so you don't have to think about it in case something happens. People tell me,

"Well it's right in my cell phone." But I always encourage keeping a hard copy on hand. Because you won't remember all of it, and it'll make things easier.

Speaking Up

One of the hardest issues when taking care of anyone (yourself included!) is advocating for the person who is being cared for. In the next chapter, I'll talk about some approaches to doing that. ❧

CHAPTER 9

Advocacy

When you're a caregiver for a family member, one of the most valuable roles you can play is to be their advocate. Advocacy comes in many forms, whether getting the patient the right equipment or dealing with professionals, finding a silver lining in a dire situation, or evaluating advice you might be getting from friends, family, or the internet.

Negativity from Healthcare Professionals

As I've mentioned, my mother had a dense stroke and was unable to communicate verbally. When I took her out of the neurological rehab center, the speech therapist decided to give me a little talk. She told me that my mother was never going to be able to eat again, even though she had a swallow test, and we knew she could swallow safely. Her feeding tube was never going to come out, she said. She was never going to talk again. She was never going to do this again or that again. "Never, never, never," was all she could say. It was demoralizing.

In a workshop I later gave to rehab therapists, I cautioned against communicating this way. "Families need to understand reality. That's true," I told them. "And they need to understand what's involved in the care of this person now. That's also true. But when you take away every shred of hope, they can't function. You have to be able to find something that they can hang onto so they can continue caring for that person."

My response to that speech therapist was to tell her that I come from a center where we treat people with dire conditions all the time, and we always say, "We'll see." People ask things like, "Will your restorative nursing program work? Will they be able to do this or do that?" And our initial response is "We'll see. We're working on it. We'll see. No promises."

> "What can we hope for? What are some positives that we might be heading toward? What are some goals that we can work on, and how are we going to get there?"

I don't want to give false hope to people. If I know someone's paralyzed, I'm not going to tell them they're going to walk again. But we find something for the family to hold onto. Maybe we say, "Well, they're not going to be able to walk again. But we think our restorative nurses are going to be able to enable them to do this other thing again."

My advice to you in this situation is to try to get to that information. If all you're getting is negativity, ask, "What can we hope for? What are some positives that we might be heading toward? What are some goals that we can work on, and how are we going to get there?"

Don't hesitate to let your need for some positivity or to learn about small goals be known.

Organizing the Care

When you have people coming into your home to provide care for your loved one, you need to develop a method for organizing around them. I like to write things down, especially when you have multiple people providing care. Because when you have multiple people, there are too many chances for mistakes. "I didn't realize you gave him his medication already. And now I've given him his medication." Or, "I thought you were going to bathe him. He didn't get bathed." There are just too many chances for too many mistakes to be made.

To prevent confusion surrounding my husband's care, I created a form. And when anyone did something listed on the form, they initialed it and checked it off. That way, I knew and everyone else knew that it had already been done.

Having a form like this frees you from having to supervise constantly. You need to speak up only when you see something hasn't been done rather than checking with your care providers all day long.

Difficult Caregivers in Your Home

Someone I know had a series of caregivers who would come to the house to care for his wife. One of them was very bossy. She was good at feeding his wife and bathing her, but she was a difficult presence. She brought feelings of unease into the house. Everyone felt like they were walking on eggshells around her, as her responses were unpredictable.

When his daughter observed this and suggested he speak up, he urged her to keep her thoughts to herself. "Don't say anything to her because she might leave."

I had the same situation with one caregiver who took very good care of Frank. But I knew he was doing things he shouldn't be doing in my house. My son was very upset and said, "How can you tolerate him here? Get rid of him." And my response was, "Your dad is a very big guy. Finding caregivers who can physically handle him is hard. And he does take good care of Dad. I'm going to live with the rest of it."

That's what you end up doing. You end up living with a less-than-ideal situation: as long as they're taking good care of the person that they're supposed to be taking care of, you might need to live with the rest. Because finding good, responsible caregivers is hard. It might not always feel right, but if you found someone who is taking good care of your loved one, an unfortunate reality is that you might need to grit your teeth and stick with them.

Unsolicited Advice

I've covered this subject a couple of times already, but it bears repeating in the context of advocating for someone: everyone has an opinion. Everyone thinks they know what you should do.

How do you deal with these opinions that you never asked for? While you might listen to what's being said (and you might not!), in the end you need to stand your ground and do what, in your heart, you think is best.

I had a conversation with a young mother recently, who was talking to me about her daughter with mental health problems. She said, "Everyone has an opinion about what to do. My mother, the pediatrician, my next-door neighbor—everyone has something to say." But then she told me, "I've been thinking about what you said, and you're right. In my gut, this is my daughter. I know what's best for her. I know her better than anyone knows her. This is what needs to be done, and I'm going to stick to my guns and demand that they do that." And I said, "That's good. That's what you need to do."

TOO MANY COOKS

There's an old saying that too many cooks spoil the stew, meaning that too many people throwing things into the mix can ruin the taste of the stew. This principle applies to advice. It's best to identify a few people who you trust and whose advice you value. Ignore the constant flow of other opinions. Not only is it difficult when people give their opinion and make you feel unsure of yourself, it could be overwhelming to get too many opinions. Don't hesitate to politely shut people down when they volunteer an unwanted opinion. For example, you can say, "I appreciate your concern, but I have the information I need to move forward, and I'm not looking for more advice."

Where Do You Get Your Information?

To advocate for someone experiencing health or other issues, you need to be able to separate fact from fiction.

For example, I'm working on a project, a therapeutic approach for post-traumatic stress (PTS). A group of people is working on this, many of whom are not clinicians. I appreciate who they are and what they do. But I often get emails from them about new techniques for PTS. They might say, "My friend in California says this works really great."

And I ask, "Can I see the research?"

"Well, there's no research," they say. "We're dealing with anecdotal evidence."

Anecdotal evidence essentially means that someone had an experience that they told someone about. There was no methodical, reviewed study to back up any claim of effectiveness. So, I have to tell them, "I'm sorry, but the fact that your friend thought this therapy worked isn't good evidence."

If hearing about something from a friend or acquaintance isn't a good way to learn about possible therapies, how do you go about finding valid information? Searching on the internet and finding an answer on a random website or on a user forum is not the way! That approach has caused much confusion and sometimes even harm. Because you're always going to find a website that backs up a claim. "See? It says so on the internet!" you might think. But simply being on the internet is not good enough.

> 66
> Before buying into information you find online, investigate the site where you found it.

Before buying into information you find online, investigate the site where you found it. Is it a commercial site trying to sell a treatment? That's generally not a good place to learn about the validity of a therapy. If the site references a study, find the study to see if it was published in a scientific journal. You *can* rely on hospital sites, university (.edu) sites, government (.gov) sites, and well-known nonprofits associated with the condition. If you haven't heard of the nonprofit, read the About page on the site to understand the organization's charter and who is behind it.

An excellent site for understanding how to find health information on the internet is maintained by the National Institutes of Health: https://

www.nia.nih.gov/health/online-health-information-it-reliable. (The NIH itself is an excellent source for health information as well.)

Before you make changes to your loved one's health regimen based on something you read online, it's crucial that you speak with the prescribing physician. Every patient is different, and using a website to make a medical decision can be dangerous. Bring what you've learned to the practitioner and ask questions. For example, journal articles can be very hard to understand, and often their results are based on a sample that is too small to apply to the population in general. Bring articles like this to your next appointment to get a professional's input on them.

The most dangerous thing that I've seen happen multiple times is that someone looks into something on the internet, and then they act on what they found. They stop a medication, or they add a supplement that doesn't interact well with an existing medication. They might do a number of things without consulting with their practitioner. I've seen disasters happen because of that. If you stop a certain medication suddenly, for example, negative side effects can occur.

So, while I think it's important to trust yourself when advocating for a patient, if something is outside your area of expertise, you need to take what you've learned and discuss it with the professionals. Don't stop the patient's treatment plan on your own.

Wrapping Up

On my radio show, I like to end each episode with what I refer to as "takeaways." In the next, concluding chapter, I'd like to share some of those takeaways and summarize advice that's common to caregivers of people of all ages. ❧

A Few Takeaways

I've covered a wide range of issues throughout this book. I've summarized a few thoughts in the form of what I call "takeaways" in my radio show.

Your Feelings

Everyone needs to vent. When you're taking care of someone—whether raising a child or caring for a partner or parent—you are apt to feel emotions like frustration, anger, or resentment.

When you're having a rough moment, you don't want your child, spouse, or parent to know how you're feeling. However, most people have at least one trusted friend they can talk to who will not repeat what they're saying. It's okay to vent to them and get it out.

Sometimes we get very angry inside. A friend of mine used to say, "I sometimes wish we could freeze-dry the children. Then when we are ready to deal with them, we could just snap our fingers and they'd be back to normal." This desire for relief is common.

I often deal with parents who become very angry and upset with their children's behaviors. I also interact with family members who feel the same way about a senior.

I tell all of these caregivers the same thing: all of us have strong and negative feelings at times. You love your parent, your spouse, or your child, but sometimes it feels like too much. What's important, though, is what you do with your feelings.

If you're feeling out of control, take a deep breath. Step outside for a few minutes. Do something that will help you to calm down. And ask for help. Caregivers tend to do it alone, and it makes the frustration and anger even worse. It's important to have strategies that work for you when you are upset, and it's important to let people help you so that you can refuel.

Self-Talk

Words carry a lot of power. How we talk to ourselves and how we phrase our thoughts can bring us hope or bring us stress and worry. It can determine our perceptions of people and events. So, choose the words that will bring you comfort and peace.

I admire the book *The Gift of Maybe*, by Allison Carmen, which emphasizes the power of words. It includes my favorite quote from Khalil Gibran, which I previously shared in the introduction.

"Your living is determined not so much by what life brings to you as by the attitude you bring to life, not so much by what happens to you as by the way your mind looks at what happens."[5]

---

5   Kahlil Gibran, quoted in Allison Carmen, *The Gift of Maybe: Finding Hope and Possibility in Uncertain Times* (New York, NY: Penguin Group, 2014), 10.

How do you apply this quote to your own life? Think about the thoughts that go through your head while lying in your bed trying to fall asleep. Are you thinking about how your children or your father annoyed and frustrated you that day? If so, try instead being grateful that your children are healthy and safe. Try remembering the good things that your father did for you when you were a child and be grateful that you have been given the opportunity to model for your own children how to treat older parents.

Changing how you think is good for you and might even result in being able to fall asleep more quickly and to sleep more peacefully if you're stuck on negative thoughts at night.

The ways we phrase our thoughts can bring us hope and comfort or bring us stress and worry. It is your choice.

> **"**
> You need to take care of yourself so you will have the inner strength and mental stamina to continue to care for others.

Self-Care

You can't continue to do what you do without taking care of yourself. You are critical to everyone around you, and so you must become a priority. For example, getting enough sleep for yourself is just as important as it is for children.

You need to take care of yourself so you will have the inner strength and mental stamina to continue to care for others. Make yourself a priority. At some point, you have to go to the top of your to-do list. As I am fond of saying: Do just one small thing for yourself every day. Just one thing.

We consistently put many things in our life on the back burner, including time to take care of ourselves. But most of us keep some kind of schedule book, whether it's electronic or paper. Use that device to schedule time to accomplish at least one or two of those tasks that are for *you* that you have been putting off. Block out time that's for you.

One of the benefits to doing this is that you might feel a sense of accomplishment and be pleased that a burden has been lifted off your shoulders. If you have the opportunity to refuel, you've put yourself in a better position to continue to provide care for others.

Tips to Gain Control When Stressed

In all of the following suggestions, the most important thing to do is to turn off your internal conversations. Stop thinking, analyzing, and talking to yourself.

- Hide in the bathroom. This is my favorite as the bathroom is the one room in the house where people leave you alone. Keep aromatherapy soap in the bathroom. Enter, put down the lid, soap up your hands, sit down on the closed lid, close your eyes, and breathe deeply, giving yourself an aromatherapy moment. It only takes a few moments. Remember to lift the lid and flush so that no one will know what you were doing in there!

- Step outside and breathe fresh air.

- Sit down on your bed, close your eyes, and turn off your internal conversations.

- Sit in your car for a few moments when you arrive home. Do not go straight into the house.

- In work-related situations, practice mindfulness as you wait for your computer to start up.

- With your child or a senior, watch television. Sit down and watch it with them so it is a time-out for you, too. Your child, spouse, or parent will enjoy this time with you, and you get a brief rest.

- Watch an old movie, comedies like *I Love Lucy* or *Friends*, or a musical. The important thing is to be engaged. Don't use the time as an opportunity to do some work while they are in front of the television.

Dealing with a Lack of Privacy

When my husband was ill, spending time alone was not possible as there were always people in our home. On top of that, the caregivers often had to be in our bedroom through the night.

A lack of privacy and ability to spend time alone can often result in depression and frustration. I recommend getting out of the house and going somewhere you can spend some time alone. Take a walk, go to the library, take a drive, treat yourself to an ice cream cone—whatever works for you. The important thing is to go by yourself.

I also recommend that you schedule a power nap. Women especially tend to feel that if someone is in their home then they must always be busy and productive. That's not true. What you need is to be able to provide care. So, take a twenty-minute nap, which will allow you to continue to provide care. This is true even when caring for infants and young children. Their nap time can be your nap time. In the end you will be more productive and accomplish more if you're rested.

You might think, "But I can't take the time." I want to assure you that you can. Doing so will pay dividends. Just twenty minutes will make a significant difference in your mental and physical health.

Allowing Children to Fail

As we talked about in chapter 1, one of the ways you can be most helpful to your children is by allowing them to experience a degree of failure followed by learning how to recover from these failures. I mentioned this saying from an African proverb, which you can say to yourself when you begin feeling that you are taking over control of a situation for your children and not allowing them to take some risks. It is a personal mantra for parents and for grandparents.

Smooth waters do not make for good sailors.

How I interpret this quote is that all of us wish for smooth seas for our children and grandchildren. But in our hearts, we know that life has many bumps and that the waters are never smooth. A feeling of competency and trust in oneself is a result of having ridden out the storm. If you have never fully experienced the storm or rough waters, or someone else has always piloted the boat, then you won't have faith in your ability to succeed. When this happens, an individual's self-esteem can crumble quickly when they're suddenly faced with heavy seas.

The ability to experience failure and, from that failure, go on to succeed, is a gift. It grants a sense of inner pride in our own competency and the ability to manage the boat through the sea of life.

The Importance of Play

It's important to understand the value of play, not only with young children but also with teenagers and older family members.

Play helps people to do the following:

- Forget other things for a period of time.

- Relax, take a breath, and slow down for a few minutes.

- Laugh, which is one of the best exercises.

- Connect or reconnect to another person—not as a caregiver. Play can also include your spouse, who might feel left out because you are so busy taking care of others.

Children will play almost anything you want. The important element for them is that they have your attention. So, think about what you used to enjoy as a child. Teach your child or grandchild the games that you used to play. Maybe it's coloring. (Adult coloring is a current trend!) I bought a set of jacks to play with my granddaughter because I loved playing with jacks as a child. It really doesn't matter what you play.

I've had tough adolescents walk into my play-therapy room stating that they aren't children and will not play anything. Within the first session we are playing cards, using clay, and even playing with action figures.

In our hearts, we want to be a child again, if even for a few moments. Playing is fun and relates to later academic success. It also helps you to manage behavior.

In our hearts, we want to be a child again, if even for a few moments. Playing is fun and relates to later academic success. It also helps you to manage behavior.

It might come as a surprise, but play is also beneficial for seniors. After my mother's stroke, I bought her a special card holder so that she could continue to play cards, which she loved. The time playing cards with her was very special to me. It was relaxing for both of us.

As a caregiver, you're stressed and never have enough time. But a few minutes a day to reconnect through play is an investment in caring. And having fun is okay!

Solace in the Storm

In writing this book, my hope was to share my personal and professional experiences with you, the reader, in a way that would support you in your caregiving journeys. It is my deepest desire that you have found some pathways to comfort and respite within these pages. My heart goes out to you. You are not alone. ❧

Wishing you comfort, peace, and solace in the storm,

Dr. Merle Griff

Acknowledgments

To my father, Joseph Krouse, who taught me the importance of caring for everyone with whom you have a relationship and modeled how to express that care in many ways.

To my mother, Lea Krouse, who expressed care not only for her family and friends but for the community, which imparted to me the importance of community service.

To my maternal grandmother, Rose Hoffman, who was the ultimate grandmother and whose wisdom and expressions of caring I have tried to replicate in the relationships with my own grandchildren.

To my husband, Dr. Franklin Griff, whose caring meant so much to his patients, who embodied deep loyalty to his friends and family, and who patiently forgave me for the many mistakes I made while caring for him for many years.

To my brother, Dr. Neal Krouse, who could always be counted on to be there when I needed him. I will always fondly remember his support while I cared for my husband.

To Alicia Rozenbom, Diane Collum, Laura Solomin, and Susan Cohen, my friends in Ohio with whom I raised my children. Separated from our nuclear families, we became family to each other, giving support and advice that made those child-rearing years so much easier.

To my new friends in Florida who made my move there in the midst of the pandemic and the loss of my husband so much easier. Gloria and Gary Sherman made sure I was never alone during the first difficult months. Anne and Barry Leonard took me under their wing and remade me so that I could try to start living again. Irma Sanders always saw beneath the surface and was always there to provide wisdom and sage advice.

To my Ohio, Florida, and Pennsylvania friend, Lori Shaffron, who has always been there for me, especially through my caring for my mother and then for my husband.

To my colleagues and friends: Dr. Karen VanderVen, who taught me how to be a mentor; Sr. Madeleine Rybicki, whose prayers have always brought comfort; Lincoln Palsgrove, who is a trusted advisor and friend; and colleagues from whom I have learned much over the years, with a special thank-you to Candace Benson, Jed Johnson, and especially Norma Rist.

To my staff, who gave me support and stood by my side while I was a family caregiver. I could not have accomplished this and been able to care for my family without them.

A special thank-you to my executive assistant, Sheri Rimedio, whose help means so much, and to Cathy Cooke for being my wordsmith on a multitude of projects and always being there to keep me on the right path.

With deep gratitude to the members of our SarahCare family who have consistently gone above and beyond for all the families who have entrusted us with the care of their loved ones, and to our SarahCare franchisees who continue to provide the gold standard of care and who supported me in writing this book, especially all the members, both past and current, of our Franchise Advisory Council.

A special thank-you to David Webb for his unwavering dedication and support of the SarahCare mission.

To my editors and staff at Forbes Books and Advantage Media Group, your feedback and edits enhanced this book to become a significant resource in the lives of others.

With deep appreciation for Betsy Gitelman, who took my words and turned them into something special and meaningful. She has become a treasured friend through this journey.

For the never-wavering sources of delight, pleasure, and pride that are my children, Adam and Richard, and my grandchildren, Lilli and Asher. You are the loves of my life and my treasure. ❧

About the Author

Dr. Merle D. Griff, is the founder and CEO of SarahCare, an adult day health center with locations throughout the United States. She began her career working with children as a play therapist and developed therapeutic techniques that are used throughout the world. Dr. Griff brings her clinical expertise and personal experience to her podcast about caregiving throughout the life cycle, *Caught Between Generations.* ❧